NATIONAL UNIVERSITY
LIBRARY   SAN DIEGO

WHEN AUTISM STRIKES
Families Cope with Childhood Disintegrative Disorder

Edited by

ROBERT A. CATALANO, M.D.

Foreword by

FRED R. VOLKMAR, M.D.

D0557290

PLENUM PRESS • NEW YORK AND LONDON

Library of Congress Cataloging-in-Publication Data

On file

ISBN 0-306-45789-X

© 1998 Plenum Press, New York

A Division of Plenum Publishing Corporation
233 Spring Street, New York, N.Y. 10013-1578

http://www.plenum.com

All rights reserved

10 9 8 7 6 5 4 3 2 1

No part of this book may be reproduced, stored in a retrieval system, or transmitted in any
form or by any means, electronic, mechanical, photocopying, microfilming, recording, or
otherwise, without written permission from the Publisher

Printed in the United States of America

We dedicate this book in loving memory of
Daniel George Kalmer, and to all children with disabilities
and their families. May they find the happiness they deserve.

Contents

Foreword

In his classic description of the autistic syndrome, Leo Kanner (1943) originally suggested that children with autism were born with the disorder. Subsequent research has modified this impression. It is clear that most children with autism do exhibit problems in the first year or year and a half of life, but a small group of children develop autism, or something very similar to it, after what appears to be 1 or even 2 years of normal development (Volkmar, Klin, & Cohen, 1997). Of course, various factors might well act to advance or delay case detection. Some parents are more aware of what to expect from normally developing infants and note problems that other parents miss. In some cases, a child who goes on to have higher-functioning autism may speak on time but as the child develops, more unusual social behaviors or environmental responsiveness are seen. The available data do, on balance, suggest that classical autism almost never develops after 3 years of age. However, some children who develop normally for a period of several years go on to develop a clinical syndrome very similar to autism. In considering how best to classify such disorders, we must turn to the work of the special educator Theodore Heller.

Working in Vienna in the early years of this century, Heller reported on six children who exhibited severe developmental regression between 3 and 4 years of age, following a period of apparently normal development. This condition was initially termed *dementia infantilis* and, subsequently, *Heller's syndrome, Disintegrative Psychosis,* or, most recently, *Childhood Disintegrative Disorder* (CDD). In the nearly 90 years since Heller's original report, over 100 cases have been reported in the literature and the syndrome has undoubtedly been underrecognized (Volkmar & Rutter, 1995). The lack of recognition has reflected a presumption that the condition represented "late-onset" autism or was the result of the insidious onset of some progressive neuropsychological process. As a result, this condition is unfamiliar to clinicians and has only recently been recognized as an official diagnosis (APA, 1994).

Several lines of data have supported the recent recognition of CDD as a disorder apart from autism. The onset of the condition is highly distinctive and an essential feature of the diagnosis. Consistent with Heller's (1930) impression, the condition is usually observed after 3 years and before 5 years in children who previously appeared normal. The condition's onset may be abrupt (over days to weeks) or more gradual (weeks to months); sometimes there is a period of nonspecific agitation as the child begins the dramatic regression that is the hallmark of this condition.

The natural history of this condition, once established, also differs from more classical autism in that the long-term outcome is apparently *worse* than in autism. In about 75% of the cases the child's behavioral and developmental functioning deteriorates to a much lower level than in autism and then plateaus. No further deterioration occurs, but subsequent gains are minimal. In other cases, there may be some limited recovery—for example, the child may regain the capacity to speak single words. In only a handful of either of these types of cases has a child been observed to make a major recovery of developmental skills. In a small number of cases, deterioration progresses with no plateau and may result in death. These are extreme cases where the condition is of late onset and clearly associated with some known progressive neurological disorder (Corbett, 1987). Life expectancy in all other cases appears to be normal.

Given the dramatic nature of the child's regression, it is not surprising that for many years the presumption was that CDD was the overt manifestation of some *identifiable* neurological or other medical condition and, therefore, did not deserve official recognition. Again this has turned out not to be the case. Although such cases have been observed, it usually is the case that exhaustive medical evaluations do not reveal a specific medical "cause" although nonspecific abnormalities consistent with some as yet undiscovered neurobiological process or processes of seizures or abnormal brain wave activity are sometimes observed. The lack of recognition of the condition has limited research, and only now are systematic studies being conducted. Studies of epidemiology, intervention, and, of course, neurobiology are very much needed. *When Autism Strikes: Families Cope with Childhood Disintegrative Disorder* will increase awareness of this perplexing condition and, as such, can only facilitate efforts to find its causes.

This volume is a poignant testament to the enormous toll that this condition takes on afflicted children and their families. Their tremendous suffering is intensified by their experience of the children's earlier normal development, often documented in videotapes recorded prior to the regression. I applaud the courage of the families who, in this volume, eloquently provide their own accounts of coping with the human tragedy that this condition represents.

Fred R. Volkmar, M.D.
Harris Associate Professor
Child Study Center
Yale University

References

American Psychiatric Association (1994). *Diagnostic and statistical manual of mental disorders.* (4th ed.). Washington, DC: Author.

Corbett, J. (1987). Development, disintegration and dementia. *Journal of Mental Deficiency Research, 31*(4), 349–356.

Heller, T. (1930). Uber Dementia Infantilis. *Zeitschrift fuer Kinderforschung, 37*, 661–667.

Kanner, L. (1943). Autistic disturbances of affective contact. *Nervous Child, 2*, 217–250.

Volkmar, F.R., Klin A., & Cohen, D. (1997). Diagnosis and classification of autism and related issues: Consensus and issues. In D. J. Cohen & F. R.

Volkmar, (Eds.), *Handbook of autism and pervasive developmental disorders* (2nd ed., pp. 5–59). New York: Wiley.
Volkmar, F.R., & Rutter, M. (1995). Childhood Disintegrative Disorder: Results of the DSM-IV Autism Field Trial. *Journal of the American Academy of Child and Adolescent Psychiatry, 34,* 1092–1095.

Preface

This book is not for the weak of heart. To lose a child is a tragedy. To lose a child who still lives is beyond comprehension. The children chronicled in this book share a common affliction. Born healthy and happy, they lose their minds to a mysterious disorder for which there is no known cause or cure. Fortunately the disorder is rare, but more children may be affected every day, on every continent.

The book consists of eight stories of families coping with Childhood Disintegrative Disorder. The stories are of healthy toddlers plunged into a terrifying world from which they cannot escape. Collected from around the globe, the accounts are frighteningly similar. Bewildered children, old enough to recognize their world is collapsing, languish briefly on the edge of reality. Some, apparently aware of the horrid transformation occurring, plead with their parents to stop the change. Once down the abyss, most are never able to escape. Family fortunes search for causes. Consumed lives chase cures. Regrettably, this is not a horror film. It is real life.

Intent on helping their children, affected parents encounter constant disbelief from health care professionals that their children ever developed normally. They label the children "autistic" and lump them

with children who never experienced 2 to 4 years of normal development. Armed with home videos and tape recordings, advantages of the
modern age, many of the parents seek the consultation of world experts.
They press for one more test, one more chance to expose the cause.
They also try one more procedure, one more drug, and one more placement in this quest.

Why write a book? By telling stories of children with late-onset
autism, or Childhood Disintegrative Disorder, we hope that additional
children, otherwise misclassified, will be identified. A larger subset
will help researchers identify etiological and prognostic factors. The
parent authors, having endured many struggles since the onset of the
disorder in their children, also wish to share information regarding
treatment successes and failures. Finally, these parents wish to lend
support and encouragement to others in similar circumstances, as they
too cope with daily living while searching for solutions to this puzzling
disorder.

Robert A. Catalano, M.D.

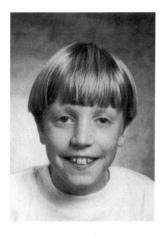

One

Per's Pages

by Kjell Berg

First Year of Life

When our son Per was born completely healthy, we experienced total happiness. It was in the middle of winter and his birth was easy, without any complications. At that time we did not know anything of the nightmare that would come 4 years later. Everything about Per was normal. He had good eye contact and smiled socially at the appropriate times. His personality was calm and pleasant.

Per said his first word very early in life. When he was 5 months old he said "eat, eat" when he wanted to be fed. The doctor had difficulty believing this, but we are certain Per had spoken the words. When Per was 1 year old he said "mother" and "father." We thought he would start talking early.

In Sweden, children take the Boel test at 8 months of age. This test determines the child's eye contact and hearing by ringing a soft bell and noting whether the child turns his head. Per was found to be "normal" by this test.

We are glad to have videotapes of Per's early childhood so we can remember how normal and happy our boy was before his regression at

1

age 4. The videotapes from this earliest period show that Per's behavior as an infant was without any abnormality.

1–2 Years Old

Although Per's development was typical, he was slightly slower than most children to learn to walk. He walked at about 19 months of age. However, Per's sister was also older than usual when she learned to walk at $17\frac{1}{2}$ months. Because she was very bright and performed at the top of her class, we thought that late walking was nothing about which to worry. Every other aspect of Per's development was absolutely normal.

Per was good at imitating our behaviors. I remember one episode when I went into the bathroom, took the scale to weigh myself, and put it on the floor. After I weighed myself, I put the scale back on the shelf. Although I was not aware that Per was watching, he had seen this episode and later did exactly the same thing.

The videotapes from this period show Per to be a very happy boy at his sister's birthday party. He walked around just like the other children with a balloon in his hand. He investigated what secrets there were in the cupboards. He talked to his mother. All of his behaviors were the same as the other children.

2–3 Years Old

At the age of 3, Per was very good at quickly putting together difficult puzzles. Even 20-piece puzzles made for children aged 3–8 were no problem for him. After Per's regression 1 year later, he had no interest in puzzles. He would hold puzzle pieces upside down, looking away with a "depressed" demeanor.

Per achieved toilet skills at age 3, as do most children. These skills he kept even after his regression 1 year later. We are thankful that when Per needs to go to the toilet, he goes himself. However, he does not verbalize this need.

The videotapes from this period show Per playing with cats and in the sand. He pretended to bake a cake while digging in the sand just like any other little boy.

3–4 Years Old

Per was a little poet. The first hot, summer day he went out into the garden wearing only his shorts. He could feel the air stream around his body, and ran about happily shouting, "I am bathing in the air."

Per could say whole sentences, and he often repeated sentences emphasizing different words. He could say a sentence 10 times, with different emphasis each time. Per did not initiate speech very often but we felt that more speech would soon come.

Until Per was $3\frac{1}{2}$ years old, he stayed at home with his mother. Once reaching $3\frac{1}{2}$, Per went to a day-care home. We did not notice any differences between his behavior and that of the other children. Perhaps Per had a little more energy. After lunch, while the other children slept, Per liked to walk up and down the stairs.

He had good eye–hand coordination. When we were in a shop and Per saw an unlocked candy pot, he raced to it, grabbed sweets, and put them in his mouth. Per was so quick that we could not stop him. He did the same thing at home when he saw a plate of cakes. First Per checked to make sure we were not watching him, then he quickly grabbed a cake and put it in his mouth so we could not take it from him. He was like a hawk that never missed its prey.

The videotapes from this period show Per riding a tricycle and a toy tractor. His speech is good and he talks about many things. Sentences such as "I want to cycle now," "I want to pat the cat," and "I want to go barefoot" are common.

It is a great mystery how a boy who seemed completely normal could undergo the personality change that Per did during his fourth to fifth year of life. We will always wonder how it could have happened. There were no illnesses, no accidents, and no other circumstances that could explain it. We have no explanation at all for Per's regression.

4–5 Years Old

At 4 years of age, Per went to the doctor for a checkup. He found Per a little different than most children and therefore performed various tests. However, no problems were found. "He is a little late in progress, but it is nothing to worry about," said the doctor.

At 4 years 3 months, Per's regression occurred. He started running back and forth and could not be calmed. He put everything in his mouth including nonfood items such as grass, gravel, stones, flowers, and once even fly agaric. (We made many telephone calls to the poison information central.) Per's talking decreased and he seemed depressed, although hyperactive. We lost contact with him. When he looked at me, I felt that he was looking through me. When I asked him something, he answered with the same question. Before his regression, Per could lay for hours on the kitchen floor drawing in his book or cutting papers. Now he could not even hold a pencil or scissors properly. When he tried to cut and found that he could not, he was so upset that he cried. In 2 weeks, Per's personality completely changed. It was so fast that the doctor suspected bleeding or a tumor in his brain. Per was immediately tested with a CT scan. Later, he had an EEG and other tests. All results were normal. Not knowing what was wrong was frustrating. The doctors said that Per's behavior resembled autism. As most parents in this situation would do, we started reading about autism. Frightfully, when we asked the doctors what we could do about it, they talked about institutions.

This period was the most difficult time in my life. We were learning about autism and at the same time trying to get Per an assistant and other help. We also had to take Per to various tests. The night before an EEG test I walked him back and forth down the hospital corridors many hours to keep him awake so he would be tired enough to sleep during the test. During the blood tests I had to use all of my strength to hold him down. However, Per was a brave little boy, and has five medals for bravery on his bedroom wall.

5–6 Years Old

During this period a strange episode occurred that I will never forget. Per had been saying only one or two words every day. He did not want to have any physical contact with us such as sitting on our laps. Suddenly one morning Per climbed up on my lap, looked me straight in the eyes, and pointed with his finger to my head. Per said, "There is an old man sitting in there." I was so surprised that I did not know what to do. I pointed to his head and asked Per if an old man is sitting in there, too. Per answered, "He sleeps." He said no more that day, but this incident made me wonder what Per was thinking about.

Per came down with scarlet fever complicated by infections in his knees and hip. He had a high fever and was in such pain that he cried whenever he was touched. He could not walk because of the pain so we had to carry him. (We knew then that Per feels pain. However, it takes more pain for him to react than for most children. When he cries he is in intense pain.) As he could not walk, Per had to tell us what he wanted. Therefore, his speech temporarily improved. It also seemed that speech came easier to Per when his fever was high.

My wife and I joined a group of parents in our town who have children with all forms of autism. Together we discussed and learned about the disorder. We studied a book written by Professor Christopher Gillberg, a leading Swedish scientist in the field. We did not know exactly what kind of autism Per had. Suddenly one evening we read about Childhood Disintegrative Disorder (CDD). We both instantly recognized all that was written. At last all of the pieces in our puzzle were in place. It felt like coming home. Per had CDD.

A huge dilemma for parents of autistic children is whether to pursue extensive medical examinations and drug treatments. Although medications may make the child better, they also may make him worse and further alter his personality. We decided that as long as there was no clear evidence of a medication that would make Per better, we would not pursue drug treatments. We did not want to risk the small improvements Per had already gained. As we now knew that Per had CDD and had tested him in so many ways, we did not think that he needed any more medical examinations. Instead we tried to provide Per with as much family time as possible. My wife was born on a farm in the countryside near our town. She now had bought the farm from her parents, and we tried to be there as often as possible. Per was very pleased to be there and climbed the stones that his mother also had climbed. We also walked in the forest where we could see elk and deer. It was paradise for Per, and we did not need to worry about traffic and other city dangers. Outside the house, Per could walk and explore wherever he wished.

While inside the house, Per sat on the kitchen table every day for 4 months, hitting the chairs. It was very frustrating because the chairs fell to the floor with noise heard throughout the house. We tried everything to stop Per from sitting on the table but nothing worked. After 4 months Per suddenly stopped sitting there, and has never done so again.

Someone has said that after they had seen the movie *Rain Man,* they tried to get their child used to different methods of transportion, so we also decided to take Per traveling using different methods of transportation so that he would become accustomed to them. We decided to fly to Madeira. We were fearful of how Per would react to being high in an airplane. Several months earlier we had been in a high tower when Per suddenly became terrified as he looked down. "Falling down it," Per had cried. We need not have worried about this airplane trip. On the contrary, Per was very angry and cried when we landed in another airport after 45 minutes and we had to leave the airplane. He cried the whole hour we were on the ground and did not become calm until we boarded the airplane again. When we were back home, we asked Per how it felt to fly on an airplane. He sat silently, pondering the question for a long time, and then suddenly he said "Sit down!" We laughed when we realized he had heard that phrase from us on the airplane!

The journey to Madeira and a year later to the Canary Islands appeared beneficial for Per. It is easy to travel with Per as he enjoys riding in buses or cars, and he sleeps well in different locations. The most difficult part of traveling with Per is eating in restaurants. He wants to look at everything and run around while he eats. This problem is solved by eating in hotel rooms when traveling.

6–7 Years Old

We discovered that Per could say complete sentences on two different occasions. The first was when he really wanted something. He said sentences such as "Do you want to take me out?" and "Can I have a cake?" The other occasion was when Per was surprised. One incident can explain this. Per was often so hyperactive that he could not fall asleep. He jumped on his bed shouting "iiiiiiii!" After 2 hours of listening to his shouting we were tired and lay down beside Per to try to put him to sleep. Of course I fell asleep but not Per. Suddenly he jumped up shouting "iiiiiiii!" right into my ear. I woke up and yelled "Now you must sleep!" Per immediately said, "You must not shout so, Dad!" After that sentence, Per spent 2 more hours shouting "iiiiiiii!" and jumping, before falling asleep. Per also said an appropriate spontaneous sentence one day while walking by the television. A film from Africa was being shown of a lion who had caught a zebra. "Oh, he ate it!" Per exclaimed.

Per has a good memory. At times he has suddenly started talking about things that happened years earlier. One occasion that apparently made an impression on Per was an outing on the ice with his uncle. He spoke about this day 2 years after it occurred. Another notable topic was the illness of a neighborhood boy. Per talked about this 3 months later.

When Per was 6 years old, his gross motor coordination was good. He learned how to ride a bicycle. Per also learned to jump on one leg and could hop this way for half an hour. We could not stop him! We were very grateful for Per's every improvement.

There were two situations that caused trouble between Per and his older sister. One conflict resulted from Per putting everything in his mouth and then chewing. He took his sister's possessions such as pencils and chewed them up. Besides destroying her things, Per woke up early on weekends and ran around shouting, thereby preventing his sister from sleeping. Otherwise, Per and his sister got along quite well. She often took Per outside and played with him. When her friends came to visit, they all played with Per.

7–8 Years Old

Per's swimming skills progressed to the point where he could swim more than 25 meters. At first he would not dip his head under the water but after this happened accidentally, Per realized he could hold his breath and started swimming under water like a fish. We are glad that Per enjoys swimming with us as a family activity.

At 7 years of age Per began school. He went to a special school and was in a class with other autistic children. Per enjoyed school and his teachers were helpful and interested in teaching him. They used the

TEACCH method. Luckily, I did not have to fight to get Per assistants and extra help. It was arranged for him to have a one-on-one teacher at school and an assistant after school for his spare time.

The shock we experienced when Per suddenly got CDD made us want to help other parents in this same situation. We hoped to make this heartbreaking time easier for others. After searching for other parents of CDD children, we are now in a group of 20 similar families. Our common experience with CDD has made us lifetime friends with these families. Last year our CDD group had a meeting during which we received lectures from well-known doctors and teachers in Sweden. We discussed common behaviors exhibited by our CDD children and the doctors promised to start a research project on CDD. It is our hope that this project will help find a solution for CDD.

At the meeting it was enjoyable to watch our CDD children together at a playground. Although they did not interact with each other, they looked at each other with some level of awareness. One child giggled, one played in the sand, and one climbed. However, when one child left his area, another child went to the vacated area. It seemed like they had "contact in the isolation." This summer our CDD group will meet again and continue to share ideas about treatments for CDD.

The familes in our CDD group have some experiences in common with typical autistic children's families. One example is eating disorders, which range from a child eating only one type of food to eating everything without stopping. Per eats just about everything although his favorite food is spaghetti of which he will eat as much as possible. Once I made spaghetti mixed with spinach. It was green and Per could tell the difference at once. He refused to eat it. Per also will not eat in rooms that have many people, such as restaurants, because of the noise level and distractions.

Another commonality with autistic children's families is strained relationships between extended family members. In our CDD group there are couples who have lost contact with their parents or siblings because of having a child with CDD.

Although some autistic children exhibit exceptional skills such as memorizing telephone directories, in our CDD group we have not found such abilities except for musical skills. Of course our group is only a small sample of the CDD population. Perhaps if we investigated a larger group of CDD children, exceptional abilities might be found.

8–9 Years Old

This summer seemed to be a hard time for Per. He had many tantrums or "hysterical attacks." We did not know why these occurred. At times Per pressed his nails into our skin in desperation deep enough to cause bleeding. However, Per has never shown any self-injurious behaviors.

Per has knowledge of the concepts "color," "days," and "age" but has difficulty answering specific questions correctly. When asked what color something is, Per always answers with the name of a color, but usually it is not the correct color. He knows the names of all of the days in order, but when asked what day it is he usually answers "Thursday." If you tell him it is the wrong answer, he guesses another day. When asked how old he is, Per always says "6 years old." He learned his age when he was 6. It is difficult for Per to change something he has learned.

9–10 Years Old

Per had a good year with some behavioral improvements and academic progress. His "hysterical attacks" ceased. At school he continued to be taught skills needed to lead as normal a life as possible. Per's typical daily schedule is as follows:

06:45–07:30	We wake Per up and he eats breakfast
07:30–08:00	The taxi comes and drives him to school
08:00–13:00	School
13:00–16:00	Per's assistant takes him to spare time activities
16:00–17:00	We take Per out for a daily walk, an activity he really enjoys
17:00–21:30	At home
21:30–06:45	Bedtime and Per sleeps until morning

It is important for Per to have consistent structuring of his days. We try to do the same thing at the same time every day. If we eat supper at 19:00 every day, then Per knows soon it will be bedtime even if he has difficulty understanding the time schedule. When he has a holiday, we try to keep the same time schedule as if he were at school. It is easier for Per to resume school after a holiday if he stays accustomed to a schedule.

As Per will most likely outlive us, he must be prepared for eventually living without us. We have Per spend some holidays and weekends in a special home, to be accustomed to sleeping away from home and interacting with people other than teachers and family members.

It is easiest for Per to learn in real-life situations, and when he is happy and motivated to learn. Therefore, we often teach Per while he is performing enjoyable activities such as biking, swimming, or walking with our family. One example of how this learning style is beneficial occurred when we taught him the difference between left and right. It appeared useless to teach Per this concept while he was sitting in a chair. However, when we bicycled with Per and told him to "turn left" or "turn right," he could see the difference and reap the benefit of this knowledge.

Per understands much of what we say to him. He has also demonstrated comprehension of what we have said to each other even when we spoke in complex sentences. Per follows many one step directions such as "take your jacket."

Unfortunately, Per has not progressed in speech since his regression. He usually says only single words. We use a computer with speech to teach him to say words. It seems easier for Per to repeat words the computer says than words people say to him.

Per is very musical. After he hears melodies one time, he can sing them. Even complicated melodies such as demonstrations on the keyboard, he repeats correctly. When Per hears a tune on the radio, he will continue singing it once the radio is turned off. Per often walks around while singing songs. Presently his favorite tune is *She Loves You* by the Beatles.

So far Per has not shown any interest in learning how to count, read, or write. However, he seems more interested in learning letters this year. Per has regained some of his puzzle skills even though he performed better when he was 3 years of age.

It is difficult for us to know what Per can and cannot do because he does not understand how to verbalize his knowledge to us. Per appears to know much more than we realize. He communicates his knowledge to us with actions rather than words. For example, we did not know that Per knew how to start a car. He likes to ride in the car, and one day he got in the car before we were ready to leave. After waiting a while for the others, Per became impatient to go riding so he put my hand on the ignition key and twisted it around to show me how I should start the car so we could get going!

10 Years Old

As Per has recently celebrated his 10th birthday, it seems appropriate to summarize our feelings about CDD. Even though our daughter says everything is fine and she has nice times with her friends, we realize that she is not experiencing a "normal" childhood. Therefore, we make an effort to spend as much time as possible with our daughter to show her we care for her even though we are busy with Per. One of us plans to take her on a special trip to Disneyland Paris (which would be difficult for Per to attend given the level of sensory input there). As siblings are the closest relatives to a child with CDD, and will probably outlive their parents, these siblings may one day have the responsibility of caring for the child with CDD. Because this knowledge must place great pressure on siblings, we feel it is beneficial to let our daughter take part in discussions and decisions involving her brother with CDD.

We are now used to CDD. Life has to go on. Presently Per's life is peaceful. His behavior is calm with no "hysterical attacks" and he is making small but steady academic progress. We know that the more Per learns, the better will be the quality of his life. Therefore, we must teach him as much as possible while giving him a childhood as pleasant as possible.

No one knows what the future will bring or whether Per will ever become free of CDD. We love our son with CDD very much. However, we are grateful for the memories of spending Per's first 4 pre-CDD years together and miss the Per who once was, and still is there somewhere deep inside. I as a father have a dream that I someday can continue this chapter with a complete book on Per's life. I hope I can title it: "The boy who was born twice."

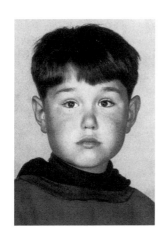

Two

Pickle

by Sheila Brown

My Brother

My brother looks like any other 7 year old brother. He is 137 cm tall and weighs about 30 kgs. He even looks a bit like me, except he is shorter and a little wider. Like any 7 year old, he loves riding his bike, swimming, jumping on the tramp and watching cartoons on TV. At the moment his favorite activity is cycling over to the neighbors and raiding their biscuit tin. Unfortunately he is not a very good burglar, because he leaves a trail of biscuit crumbs on the floor. He knows all about cars. For example, he knows you have to fill the petrol tank up with water from the garden hose. And if anyone is silly enough to leave the keys in the ignition, he will drive the car through the garage wall. In fact, he is a specialist mechanic, at least he can take things apart, but he is not so good at putting them together again. He can speak well too, but this is where it gets strange. You see, we don't always understand what he is talking about and he can't answer questions.

He is a happy boy some of the time. He sings and dances, but it doesn't take long to work out that he is different. Peace and quiet never last long in our house. We never take him on holiday, because people think he is badly behaved. You see, my brother is special. He has always been special, but now he has special needs too. When he was 4, something went wrong with his brain. Now it does not work like other people's. If anyone asks, we say he is autistic.

—*From a school speech by Andrew Brown, age 12*

The Good Old Days

"I am afraid the result is positive," said the nurse sympathetically. She was assuming that two apparently geriatric adults would not want another baby!

Stew, my husband, and I were overjoyed. At the age of 34, and after 2 years of hoping, we were at last expecting another child. Persistent and extensive nausea tempered our joy a bit, but that would pass once the baby was born. Anyway, the nausea was a positive sign that the pregnancy was progressing well.

At 15 weeks, I went for a scan. I casually asked the technician if there was more than one baby. I had been taking Clomid, a fertility drug, and there was also a history of twins in my family. She assured me there was only one.

A few minutes later, she grabbed my arm and said in a surprised voice, "I've just found another little one!" Then, a few seconds later, she pleaded "Don't tell anyone I told you, we are not supposed to tell patients anything. They can be a bit funny around here!" We were even more overjoyed to be expecting twins. We had always wanted more than two children and time was fast running out.

My twin pregnancy progressed smoothly, apart from extreme nausea and vomiting, which lasted for 7 months. At 20 weeks, I was sent to hospital for bed rest. I spent a week there before Stewart's mother, Barbara, came to our rescue. She came and stayed with us on our farm, close to Lake Taupo, in the central North Island of New Zealand. She did a great job looking after Stew and our son Andrew, then 4 years old. This allowed me to continue with "bed rest" at home. Stew and I very much appreciated all of the effort and sacrifices Barbara made on our behalf.

We knew the birthday of our expected twins long before they arrived. Having already had a Cesarean with our older son, Andrew, the theatre was booked for an elective Cesarean on Tuesday, August 13, 1985, when the babies would be 38 weeks.

When the day arrived, I was given an epidural and strapped to the operating table with a screen across my chest. Stew sat beside me wearing a gown and white gumboots. A red line was drawn on my stomach, the incision was made, and the buckets were filled. At 9:25 AM, Katie was brought into the world yelling her head off. She was a chubby 6-lb 9-oz bundle with an Apgar of 8/9. (Apgar is the responsiveness test used as a routine check on all new babies; the maximum score is 10.) Nicky followed a few minutes later. He looked wide eyed, but was very quiet and a bit scrawny. He was bigger boned than Katie, but only weighed 5 lb 13 oz. Obviously, he had been the second one on the feed line. However, his Apgar was 9/10. Despite his disinclination to suck for a couple of days, he was soon making rapid progress. Within 2 weeks of coming home from the hospital, he had put on 2 lb.

Both Katie and Nicky continued to make good progress. It was obviously tiring having two babies at once, but Stew was a great help, and most of the time both seemed to realize that it was a waste of breath to cry when the other was crying or being attended to. In fact, they were generally much more settled and less demanding than their older brother, Andrew, had been at the same age. Perhaps Andrew had played on the luxury of being an only child. The twins were rarely ill, apart from an occasional cold. They reached all of their milestones within age-appropriate times. Meanwhile, they began to develop their own unique personalities. We dubbed Katie "the schoolmarm." She often had a slightly prim, disapproving look on her face, and always seemed to know exactly what she was doing. Nicky was much more happy-go-lucky and often seemed to get himself in a muddle. Hence his nickname, "Pickle." Otherwise, they were known as the cabbage patch twins, after the dolls of the same name who were just as rotund.

In 1986, livestock prices were low, so we didn't put the ram out to the ewes on our sheep farm. This meant that for once there were no young stock to tend to on the farm. We decided to take the opportunity to visit my family in England. Traveling 12,000 miles with two 15-month-olds who had just started to walk independently was not a task everyone would choose, but we managed. It was probably made easier by the fact that I purposely did not stop breast-feeding until after we returned. I still remember Katie sucking for 6 hours nonstop between Singapore and Auckland. Every time I tried to dislodge her, the resultant yells were too much to bear.

Just before Katie's and Nicky's second birthday, I started taking them to the local playcenter once a week. It was a stimulating outing for all of us, and I soon became the principal of the center. This job lasted for 3 years, until Katie and Nicky started school. Of necessity, we attended occasions with many other children and their parents. There was never any question that Nicky was anything but normal until he was at least 4 years old.

At the age of 3 years 9 months, Katie and Nicky also started attending the local state "kindy" (preschool) in nearby Taupo, twice a week. Although Nicky and Katie played well together, I thought they would benefit from extra association with other children. Throughout this period, they both continued to develop in tandem. Sometimes Katie was ahead, at other times Nicky. Both developed good language, and they played together imaginatively. Nicky had a quirkier personality than Katie. He had a great sense of humor and laughed easily. He loved going out on the motorbike around the farm with Stew. He preferred playing with mechanical toys, dismantling them and putting them together, rather than using pen and paper. But isn't that typical of many boys? However, one memory in particular stands out. Nicky, aged 18 months, fell backward into a rose bed, and Katie anxiously came running for help to rescue him. A couple of weeks later, Katie fell in exactly the same way. Despite her yells, Nicky just sauntered past and showed no concern at all. We attributed the different reactions to maternal instinct on Katie's part, but maybe Nicky's self-centered actions were a portent of things to come. Both Nicky and Katie have always been healthy children. Apart from minor coughs and colds, Nicky was the only one to have slight medical problems. He suffered from persistent mild eczema and mild diarrhea for many years. At age 30 months, he even had the distinction of voiding blue-green feces after eating a blue-green ice cream cone.

We used to joke about Nicky's sluggish nervous system. From around the age of 3 years, we noticed his slow reaction to pain. A fall or a tap on the leg did not evoke as speedy a reaction as at a younger age. In retrospect, this was our first inkling that something was not quite right.

In New Zealand, children are entitled to a free health check done by the local Public Health Nurse around their fourth birthday. I took Katie and Nicky for theirs about 3 months after their fourth birthday. Both were put through their paces and received a clean bill of health. I was concerned that Nicky's language development was not keeping up with Katie's. However, I was assured that his language was well within the normal range and that as a twin and a boy I should expect him to be a bit behind.

The Decline

We went home and put the worry out of our minds. Soon afterward, however, a friend from the playcenter, who often had Nicky to her house to play with her children, mentioned that on occasion Nicky seemed to be unduly agitated. We had noticed this too, but what could we do? Following these periods, he seemed to have phases of "not being with it," isolating himself from what was going on around him. These periods did not last long, but long enough to disturb us. Unfortunately, over the next few months, these incidents became gradually more pronounced. We assumed he was going through some strange developmental glitch. We thought we might be putting him under too much pressure, so around Easter we stopped taking him to Kindy. He just went to the playcenter twice a week. This seemed to help, although I was sufficiently worried to approach Nicky's prospective teacher to voice my concerns.

Our next worry surfaced in May 1990 when Nicky sometimes did not respond to our voices. Tests revealed he had glue ear, and medication was prescribed. What a relief! Nicky's glue ear disappeared, but his apparent lack of hearing did not improve. We visited the ear, nose, and throat specialist, and learned that Nicky had perfect hearing. All of this just seemed so strange; it was beyond our understanding. Better to just ignore the problem and it will go away, or so we thought.

Nicky and Katie started school on August 13, 1990, their fifth birthday. Using a simple comprehension test, Nicky was assessed as having a mental age of over 6 years. We breathed a sigh of relief again. I thought Nicky was probably going to be dyslexic (as his father is). We knew dyslexia to be a relatively minor problem. Nicky still was not very interested in using pen and paper, but he enjoyed stories and could draw at an age-appropriate level.

Around this time, two close neighbors developed very severe back problems. Another lady, two houses away, developed lupus, and her husband's sight mysteriously deteriorated. All of these people were in their early 40s or younger. Many others in our community were also having problems. The farming industry was depressed. We felt very fortunate; we had a healthy family and Stew was very successful. We had an attractive home and were without money worries. I began to feel it was all too good. It felt as if something should go wrong, but even then we had our blinders on. It never occurred to us that Nicky would be our bombshell. Despite our worries, Nicky seemed to settle into school quite well. Myra, his very dedicated teacher, thought he was a bit strange but not abnormally so. Nicky's first report, written 4 months after starting school, described him as "speaking well most of the time, taking part in group discussions, but sometimes needing time to order his thoughts." The report also mentioned that "he can hear well, but if preoccupied does not always respond." He was progressing steadily through the emergent reading skills, and seemed to understand all basic concepts in math but took time to "verbalize." The report also said that Nicky was "very interested in all that goes on around him and has friends, but often prefers to play alone." Finally the report noted that "Nicky puts a lot of effort into physical education, and he is happy and well mannered." Despite our blinders, one thing worried me. Throughout this period, Nicky had periods of talking nonstop gibberish. He spoke readily, and what he said was grammatically correct, but we could not make sense of it. Our lack of understanding did not seem to bother Nicky. Our occasional "yes" or "is that so" was enough to keep him talking. Another characteristic that was creeping into his language was "perseveration" (although I had not known this term then). Nicky started to verbally fixate on certain topics, sometimes for several days.

There was no doubt about it, something strange was happening, but we still had our blinders on. Anyway, who ever heard of a perfectly normal child 5 years old becoming "queer in the head"?

Nicky continued to act in a peculiar fashion throughout the Christmas holidays. In particular, he started having difficulty falling asleep. He also began to become anxious in new situations; he refused to leave the car anywhere other than at his own home. The final straw occurred in late February. Nicky suddenly became convinced that he was a "mean Maori" (the Polynesian people of New Zealand). As such, he had to destroy the toy boat his brother, Andrew, had painstakingly been building. Nicky was beyond reason. We could no longer go on pretending that Nicky was suffering from some developmental glitch.

The Medical Trail and Speech Problems

We took Nicky to the local general practitioner (GP), and for the first time, we were forced to face the possibility of a degenerative disease. Up until then, I knew nothing of conditions such as mucopolysaccharidosis and lipidoses, but now I am all too familiar with them. This was the start of our frustrating and heartbreaking journey through the medical world. Three months later, a battery of tests, sojourns at two separate hospitals, and consultations with numerous specialists, including the highest in the land, resulted in no clear diagnosis. The term *acquired expressive/receptive language dysphasia* was mentioned. Childhood Disintegrative Disorder/Disintegrative Psychosis was disregarded as purportedly Nicky had not deteriorated enough. The only test that indicated any abnormality was Nicky's EEG (electroencephalogram). This revealed abnormal, but not epileptiform, brain waves that were especially pronounced in both temporal lobes. This, in conjunction with Nicky's increasingly autistic behavior, led to a tentative diagnosis of Landau–Kleffner syndrome (LKS). This is a very rare condition, best described as a kind of epileptic aphasia. Sufferers may exhibit a kind of mild epilepsy. They lose the ability to speak, often becoming quite autistic, but retain a normal nonverbal IQ.

During these 3 months, Nicky's behavior became increasingly weird. Initially, we suspected he was hallucinating. One night he was very distressed and would not fall asleep because he had "snakes" in his bed. The next morning he came to our room carrying the "snakes," popped them in our bed and happily hopped in beside them. Ten days later Nicky still had "snake" problems. On this occasion, he awoke at 12:30 AM with snakes in his bed. As fast as we "removed" them, he would find another. There was very little sleep for us that night. By daylight they did not seem so threatening. He again brought them to our bed. When asked, he said they were black and white striped. He proceeded to have his bath with them, as well as his breakfast, and they were still accompanying him at school at lunchtime.

Another strange incident occurred while Nicky was in the hospital. From his window, he was watching men digging up the road below. Suddenly, he became inconsolable. When asked what was the matter, he said, "Those men aren't doing it right, they are not doing it how I told them to." Another time at home he suddenly became very angry and tearful for no apparent reason, repeating, "They have killed my finger; it has gone blue." He then punched and pulled at his fingers, bent them back, and bit them until they bled.

We noticed too that he sometimes took a dislike to the radio or TV and would punch at them for no apparent reason, saying phrases such as "the TV is killing my songs" or "punching my shadow." We wondered if he found the disembodied nature of the voices, particularly on the radio, frightening.

Whether he was hallucinating or whether this was just our interpretation of his inexplicable language, we will never know. This strange phase of his language deterioration lasted about 18 months. His language was still grammatically correct and clearly enunciated, but often not related to anything we could comprehend. It often contained negative connotations, such as "die," "kill," or "dead meat." We could not understand the latter because he had not been exposed to any situation where these words were used. I remember many occasions when he became very angry and tearful. Once he started to throw the kitchen mop around, wailing "I had killed the floor mop" and "it [the floor mop] should be growing younger." During the latter part of this stage, he hated being undressed. He would complain that we were taking his skin off. His clothes had to be forcibly removed by two people; he would fight all the way! If at all possible, he would strip off the new clothes and put the original ones back on. He would do this even to the extent of taking the dripping old clothes out of the washing machine.

Nicky still had quiet periods when he would not respond. At other times, he would not keep quiet. One particular occasion was most memorable. We were driving home from Auckland, a 3-hour journey, and the entire time Nicky chattered *nonstop*. He spoke mostly about nasty animals and how he would kill them. For the last 10 minutes of the journey, he repeated just one word, up, up, up, up. . . ."

Speaking of "nasty" animals, Nicky also developed an inexplicable fear of most animals. A visit to the zoo was a horrendous experience. Walking past the camel was an impossibility. This fear even extended to the docile sheep and lambs that he had grown up with, as well as other mobile "animals" such as cars. Trying to cross the road was a nightmare.

This stage was probably the hardest for us. It was so frightening and inexplicable. His moods varied rapidly and for no apparent reason. Sometimes he was happy and giggly and at other times he appeared very tired, pale, and befuddled. The worst time was when he was miserable and cried for hours and hours. I remember one night in September 1991, when he cried nonstop between 9 PM and 2 AM, all the time reciting "30 days hath September" with incredible pathos. Nothing we could do would help and after a while we were too exhausted to try very much. Almost as bad were the times he became agitated and angry. During these periods he seemed to just get a buzz in his head; he would go berserk, and scream and kick for hours. We did not know what to do, and no one seemed able to help us.

The strangest thing was that he still had lucid periods when he spoke coherently and could answer questions logically. We used to liken him to a radio with erratic reception. All of his moods varied in length, sometimes minutes, sometimes hours, and occasionally days. He was unpredictably unpredictable. More disconcertingly, we believed Nicky knew something was happening to him. We sensed that Nicky knew he was losing his grip on reality. The deterioration in his language was matched by a deterioration in his intellect and behavior. An IQ test in April 1991 suggested that his ability was now in the dull normal range. It was shortly after this test that Nicky finally lost his ability to write or draw. His ability to draw had been deteriorating for several months. Although he appeared able to start a drawing quite well, he never knew where to stop. If he was drawing a person, the head would be all right but by the time he reached the feet, he would not stop. The toes would go round and round the page. Nicky's nadir occurred during June to September 1991. It was very hard for us to cope during this time. I remember him behaving so badly during the July school holidays that I was compelled to contact the local school advisory service. I wanted to know the laws regarding educating seriously disturbed children. I was certain the school would expel him when he began running away down the main road during school hours. I remember thinking of building a padded room for Nicky, as the only means of maintaining our sanity.

All of these feelings were enhanced by the apparent inactivity and lack of interest of the specialists during this stage. Prior to this, we had nothing but praise for the medical profession. We had been impressed by the speed at which Nicky had been admitted to hospital and by the thorough analysis and ancillary care he was given. Once all of the easy steps had been taken, however, the doctors' priorities took them elsewhere and we seemed to be left totally alone to cope with an increasingly distraught child.

Such apparent disinterest did little to alleviate our worries about the depths to which Nicky might deteriorate or whether his illness might ultimately be fatal. We still very much hoped he would be cured.

After reading Nicky's medical file and noting a glancing comment that Nicky might have LKS I decided to learn all I could about the condition. I spoke to Nicky's specialist and was told that the syndrome was very rare. There had been a few papers about it in the 1970s, but a literature search found little else. I wrote to the IHC Library in Wellington, and on July 20, 1991, received a copy of a paper from ARI (the Autism Research Institute in San Diego) dated 1991, giving a detailed account of LKS. More significantly, it discussed a possible surgical cure. Over the next few weeks, I collected much more information on LKS, from various American and English sources. During this time, nothing was being done by Nicky's doctors. In late July, I informed them about another suggested cure for LKS, which involved high-dose steroids. Purportedly these had to be started as early as possible after the onset of symptoms. Again, nothing happened. On August 13 (Nicky's sixth birthday), I received information from an LKS support group in the United States. Included were copies of many more papers on the subject, with further details on LKS, how to confirm it, and possible cures. I surmised that there was an excellent chance that Nicky had this condition, and moreover, *time was very critical in effecting a successful cure.* I was ecstatic. At last, nearly 2 months after Nicky was discharged from the hospital, I had all of the information that was necessary for Nicky to be treated. However, my trust that the doctors had my son's best interest in mind was severely reduced. I, with my limited resources and time-consuming methods, had discovered all of this information before any of the doctors, and they had access to a medical library on the campus.

The above is actually an edited portion of a five-page letter I wrote (but never forwarded!) to the medical complaints authority. Our distress at Nicky's condition was compounded by the fact that I had apparently found a cure, but could not persuade the specialists to perform the necessary test (a sleep-deprived EEG). This could confirm that Nicky had LKS and enable us to proceed with the cure.

We desperately hoped Nicky had LKS; it was our only glimmer of hope. At least there was a possibility of a cure, either steroids or brain surgery. To the latter end, we even contacted the surgeons in Chicago who were performing the surgery, and discussed bringing Nicky there. We eventually did get the sleep-deprived EEG, but not without a great deal of persuasive effort and further anguish. It is hard to convey the degree of powerlessness and frustration we felt. There was no conclusive evidence that Nicky had LKS. Nonetheless, we knew that some children were being diagnosed with LKS, even though their EEGs do not show the typical spike/wave pattern considered necessary for the diagnosis. Much against the advice of some doctors, Nicky was started on steroids in early October that year. The course lasted 3 months. The most obvious result was that his weight increased from 23 kg to 32 kg. In many ways, this time period was a turning point. While Nicky was on the steroids, he became much calmer. There was less undercurrent of anxiety and he was more manageable. Although he spoke less, what he said was more appropriate. In retrospect, these changes probably had nothing to do with the steroids. Rather, we were more likely witnessing the natural progression of his condition.

We visited Nicky's pediatrician on December 6, 1991. His attitude was less than helpful. He could not "justify" doing any further tests that might indicate a fatal disease. He commented, "We've done all we can, we'll just wait for his motor coordination to go, and then we'll know we can't do anything more." With comments like these, it is no wonder people lose faith in the medical profession and try other avenues. There would be no more trips to *that* pediatrician.

The Alternative Route

Whereas 1991 was the most horrific year in our lives, 1992 was the period of adjustment. Having no real diagnosis and feeling negative toward the medical profession, we decided to investigate alternative medicine. I had previously tried giving Nicky vitamin and mineral supplements, especially vitamin B$_6$, magnesium, and dimethyglycine, as suggested by Dr. Bernard Rimland and others. Although in the past these supplements did not appear to make any significant difference, we were open to new ideas.

The alternative practitioner we chose was a medical doctor. He came with rave reviews. His diagnosis, obtained by obscure kinesiological methods (involving raised arms and clutched vials), was paraquat poisoning accompanied by allergies to dairy products, corn, onions, oats, tartrazine, and chlorine. White flour was said to be particularly problematic. We did not lend much credence to the paraquat theory, as on our initial visit Stew was also diagnosed as being sensitive to paraquat, but on our second visit he had no such reaction. Nonetheless, my search for a cure had led me to discover that dairy products have been implicated in some cases of autism, and Nicky was definitely "autistic" by this stage. So we began 6 months with no dairy products, lots of pineapple juice, and attempts to find a palatable form of soy milk.

Entering the arena of allergies is an absolute mine field. There are rotation diets, elimination diets, and allergies that come and go. We investigated all. In the midst of this, our confusion was anything but alleviated by the results of a hair analysis conducted by another GP with alternative leanings. This analysis suggested that Nicky was allergic to milk and food colorings as before, but also sugar, potatoes, and tomatoes. (In late 1994, we took Nicky to another GP with similar leanings. He informed us Nicky was only allergic to cane sugar!)

For several months I tried to make bread and cakes with soy, rice, or potato flour, at great expense, and with varying degrees of palatability. In the end, we felt the trouble outweighed the results. Nicky did improve during this stage, he became more settled, but he also became more distant and often did not appear to recognize us. Again, it was probably just a phase of his condition.

It is obvious reading through my diary that at this stage we were still looking for signs of improvement in his condition. Any little improvement lifted our hopes, which were only to be dashed at a later time.

My diary is replete with anecdotes, some of which have already been mentioned. Another little gem follows: The GP who arranged for the hair analysis also suggested that Nicky have a 5-hour glucose tolerance test. I booked this at a local medical lab. When the day came, however, Nicky was in less than a cooperative mood. In other words, he screamed constantly. The doctor in charge could not wait to be rid of Nicky. He eventually suggested, very rudely and dismissively, that Nicky looked perfectly all right and if we were worried we should take him to a pediatrician!

This highlights a monumental problem that parents with children like Nicky have to face. He looks so normal that most people assume that there is nothing that a jolly good spanking would not cure. I remember one occasion, as my 38-kg son lay screaming and kicking on the pavement outside the local post office, being offered an umbrella by an elderly pedestrian with which to beat him!

Many times I have thought of getting Nicky a T-shirt printed with the words, "Don't look at me like that—my brain doesn't work like yours." Being accompanied by a 10-year-old who behaves like a terrible toddler does not do one's social life much good. We endured this for several years, either because we did not realize there were alternatives or because we were not ready to use them.

To get back to the allergy connection, one interesting development did arise from my investigation. Having made contact with Allergy Induced Autism, a group in the United Kingdom, I was able to have a sample of Nicky's urine analyzed at the Department of Biochemistry at Birmingham University. Several scientists there were investigating the possibility that a subgroup of late-onset autistic children had developed their condition because they have a low level of a particular enzyme called phenolsulfotransferase-P. Nicky's urine showed a very low level of sulfate, strongly suggesting a lack of the previously mentioned enzyme. This was similar to the other "autistic" children tested. The physicians assume that this leads to raised levels of phenols and amines in the blood, which can provoke many of the symptoms seen in autistic children.

This is, in fact, the only test apart from Nicky's EEG that has indicated anything abnormal. Obviously, there is still a great deal of research to be done along this line. We subsequently tried to verify this result by having the tests repeated in New Zealand, but we were unable to interest anyone in this. Living in a small isolated country like New Zealand has its disadvantages, even in these days of superfast international communication. As far as I can ascertain, Nicky is the only person in New Zealand with the CDD label. I know that this is an extremely rare condition, but specialists in other Western countries are more likely to be familiar with it, and hopefully are more supportive.

Education and Related Matters

Having explored the medical possibilities, the next step was to investigate the educational options. As mentioned, Nicky was still relatively normal when he started school. It was probably comparatively easy for him to remain mainstreamed. His assessment at hospital suggested that Nicky should have 20 hours per week of teacher aide time. His teacher, Myra, however, thought she could cope fine with just 10 hours of assistance. A very able friend, Jenny, whom Nicky had known for many years, was appointed to the job.

Jenny remembers this as a very challenging time. She never knew what to expect from day to day—maybe laughter, maybe tears, anger, or frustration. To her, and all of us, it was most frustrating not being able to understand what was upsetting Nicky. She remembers one day in particular. That day Nicky continually tried to run away. He had to be forcibly returned from the school gate, only to head off again as soon as possible. After 3 hours of this, the problem was solved. Nicky was cold and just wanted to go home and get his coat!

Jenny also recalls that the smallest achievements would be tremendously rewarding. She well remembers the time Nicky eventually wrote an N for his name, after weeks of trying. She was so excited, she wanted to tell the whole world. At other times, he would demonstrate amazing feats of recall. On one occasion, he quoted figures about the number of stars in the galaxy and the distance the individual ones were from the sun. There were fun times and painful moments. His laughter and enjoyment at throwing leaves in the wind or trying to fly like a bird was fun. Trying to stop him from biting or squeezing himself was agonizing.

On the matter of education, we were very lucky. In Rotorua, our nearest major city, there is a center known as the Child Potential Unit (CPU). It was originally built as a Cerebral Palsy Unit. With that condition becoming less common, it now provides residential assessment for children with special needs. The assessments usually last 3 to 4 weeks.

During that time, the children attend the unit school and are examined by all of the appropriate specialists.

To us this had a double advantage. Besides assessing Nicky's needs, it gave us our first and very much needed break from Nicky since he became ill. A child like Nicky is not only physically and mentally wearing, but also has a very detrimental effect on family relationships. Although we were not aware of it until much later, Andrew's school work had plummeted after Nicky became ill. Katie did not seem so obviously affected, but her age may have made her more resilient. Probably, Stew found the problem the hardest to bear. For quite some time, he refused to acknowledge that there was a problem. He spent as much time as possible away from Nicky, and became irate if the subject was ever mentioned. I understand that this is a fairly common attitude, but once the problem is faced, the person concerned has to make a much larger adjustment than someone who has been adjusting to the problem all along. Consequently, once Stew accepted that there was a serious problem, he still needed many years to come to terms with it.

I remember the first occasion that Nicky was in the CPU. It was a time of amazing relief. Not having him home for five days in a row made us even more painfully aware of the stress we were under. Stew used the opportunity to go on a school camping trip with Andrew, and I spent much needed time with Katie. Both Stew and I were very aware that Katie and Andrew were losing out on a lot of experiences as a family. Having a handicapped child in fact made us a handicapped family. We wanted our children to be able to play sports, join interest groups, and have as full a life as possible. Every time opportunities arose, however, the question was, do we take Nicky and risk the consequences of his antisocial behavior, or does one of us stay home and look after our problem child?

The time away from Nicky also afforded us the chance to reassess how we were treating his condition, and fortify ourselves against the next onslaught. We had hoped that while Nicky was in the CPU, there might be some progress toward a definitive diagnosis, at least something a bit more explicit than "acquired brain disorder" or "acquired receptive and expressive dysphasia with associated behavioral problems." However, that did not happen. It is easy to put a child like Nicky into a "too difficult" basket, and save face by doing nothing. I am aware that the majority of doctors sincerely want to do their best, but like anyone else, they are not happy when they do not succeed. Such an attitude is not easy to accept, however, when one has a child suffering such devastating symptoms.

I suppose that most humans have a natural desire to categorize observations. Doing this helps us understand how different features of a disorder relate to each other. I certainly felt then, and still do now, that a label would help us to understand what was happening to Nicky. It would also be supportive to realize that we were not the only family suffering the same problem. Not many doctors appear to share this view. Those whom we encountered tended to believe that labels were restrictive and limiting. In their opinion all that needed to be done was to treat the symptoms.

The staff at the CPU did give helpful suggestions regarding Nicky's educational program, and they provided very positive support for the people working with him. Shortly after his discharge, Nicky's teacher aide hours were increased to 20 hours per week. A very structured program was created, and methods to deal with his noncompliant behavior were trialed with varying degrees of success.

My most vivid memory of Nicky at this time was his near-total lack of eye contact. We took him home from the CPU every Friday afternoon. A nurse would bring him out to us. He would walk toward us, and with absolutely no recognition, continue walking straight on by. He just did not seem to know us. Yet his behavior was always noted to be the worst on Mondays just after we brought him back. Apparently he did relate to us in some way.

Reading through the report of his time at the CPU, it is clear Nicky's behavior did not differ much from that at home. He would often cry, scream, and throw himself on the ground, calling out things such as "I'm dead, I'm dead, I can't eat anything, my legs are dying." His outbursts all had a morbid content. Sometimes they occurred for no apparent reason, but at other times after a staff member asked for compliance.

As at school, Nicky enjoyed puzzles and stories, but tended to actively object or be passively noncompliant when writing or coloring was suggested. He enjoyed physical activities such as riding a bike or swimming. He appeared to understand very simple instructions, but would often "forget" before he would finish carrying them out. It was also noted that Nicky only very occasionally intentionally used communication. He spoke mainly when he was truly motivated (e.g., "I am hungry"). However, when he was relaxed and interested, he did use some appropriate language, though at a disordered or delayed level.

Having tasted a break from Nicky, particularly in a placement we were happy to leave him, we decided to give Katie and Andrew a treat and take them to Paihia in Northland for a week. We dropped Nicky off at the CPU on the way, but the discomfort we experienced was unbelievable. We all felt incredibly guilty leaving him there; neither Katie nor Andrew uttered a single word during the 2-hour journey to Auckland. It was our first trip without Nicky. It was a turning point in our lives. We all realized that although we had desperately tried to maintain a proper family life with Nicky, it just was not working.

During the rest of 1992 and 1993, Nicky remained much the same. His understanding was limited and he continued to be very disturbed. Sleeping was often difficult, but we never medicated him to sleep. Starting the middle of May 1992, he seemed to be generally more settled and sociable, and started to take more interest in things around him. Looking back he was definitely over the worst, but as always, he varied unpredictably.

There are only a few medical events worthy of note during this period. During one 6-week period, Nicky developed an inexplicable and exaggerated flickering of his eyelids. The most logical explanation was that this was the result of some abnormal brain activity. On another occasion, he was put on a course of antibiotics to control an ear infection. He developed a devastating allergic reaction; great welts appeared all over his body and left him with ugly bruises. A change in antibiotics led to even further attacks. It was a month before he was back to normal. Nicky had never suffered such a reaction before, and has not taken any antibiotics since. Maybe his immune system was disturbed by his steroid therapy. During the year after he finished the steroids, Nicky suffered with many mouth ulcers and thrushlike infections.

During this time, he also acquired a second teacher aide, Chris, who became his full-time teacher aide a few months later. She developed an amazing rapport with Nicky. He loved Chris, and she adored him. They made an ideal combination. Chris's importance to Nicky was exemplified by his habit of prefacing his sentences with, "Please Chris," regardless of whom he was speaking to.

Around Christmas 1992, he learned to ride a two-wheeler without training wheels. We were all delighted with this achievement. It turned out to be a mixed blessing. With his newfound ability and increased energy, he was rarely at home. It was all right when he rode in the paddocks, but we had great difficulty keeping him off the road. Worse, he had absolutely no road sense. Luckily, we live on a gravel road with very little traffic. More than once a disgruntled driver reported having to drive around a child sitting in the middle of the road. Short of building a high electrified fence around our property, there was no way to keep Nicky off the road. We spent many hours wondering how to keep him off the road. Just as we arrived at a plan, the problem solved itself. Nicky lost interest in going on the road. This was typical of many of the problems we had to face that year. He would develop an aberrant behavior and repeat it continually. When we finally contrived a way to control the behavior, a different problem would develop. Associated with his bike-riding stage, he started wandering over to the neighbors and helping himself to biscuits out of their biscuit jar! Luckily, our neighbors are understanding. Subsequently, Nicky's favored activity changed to walking over to another neighbor's dam, obviously a more dangerous option. Just when we were ready to electrify the gates he stopped that and started eating incessantly. Now we have locks on all of the cupboards and a padlock on the fridge!

The worst problem arose in 1994, while he was on a short course of haloperidol (given to try to make him more manageable during a very unsettled stage). It may have been just a phase, but whatever the cause, he became incredibly sociable. His eye contact improved enormously, and he loved to cuddle. Regrettably, like a 1-year-old, he started to tweak noses, pull hair, and push people. The hair pulling was particularly bothersome, especially at school. We were worried that other parents would force us to remove Nicky from school. Fortunately, that phase disappeared after about 1 year, only to be replaced by others, such as chewing his fingernails, refusing to stay in his room until the entire house was quiet, and wetting himself! "Perseveration" was again a part of our vocabulary.

Nicky's phases were very wearing, especially because he could move so quickly. Answer a phone or go to the door and he was gone. After a second assessment at the CPU, in April 1993, we decided to seek alternative care so that we could have a more enjoyable life as a family. We eventually arranged for Nicky to attend the local children's IHC home in Taupo, which he did at irregular intervals. We found the respite very rewarding. Positive changes, though, have their downside; Nicky picked up particularly foul language and mannerisms from one of the other residents. It was time to try something else.

Fortunately, we have a cottage on our farm. In August 1994 we employed Carol to stay in the cottage and look after Nicky when we needed help. This proved to be an absolute godsend. At last, we could have a normal family life, and we could make real strides at coming to terms with Nicky's disability.

The Final Diagnosis

During most of this time we still did not have a diagnosis for Nicky. After much pressure, I eventually had Nicky readmitted to hospital in November 1993. It had been 29 months since his previous admission. He was seen by the same specialists, who noted that he had deteriorated significantly in the intervening period. He now clearly fit the diagnosis of CDD, or, as it is sometimes known, Disintegrative Psychosis. We now had our box. A box that there was about a million-to-one chance of landing in, but one in which I had long suspected Nicky would belong.

Nicky continues his education at the local primary school, where he remains the only mentally handicapped child. We consider it fortunate that Chris is still his teacher aide for 20 hours per week. We are also grateful that the majority of children behave very positively toward Nicky. Many parents have even commented that they feel his presence in the school has a beneficial effect on their children.

In the last year, Nicky has started to settle down. He has become much less stressful to manage, and seems to understand more. Although he still does not speak much, there has been a noticeable increase in his language. He is much better able to convey his needs. He is also participating much more actively in sports. Most notably, there has been a major improvement in his art. He is drawing recognizable shapes once more.

We take great pleasure in all of Nicky's little achievements. Although mentally he may only be functioning at a 3-year-old level, he is physically well coordinated and enjoys all manner of outdoor activities. He continues to have a bizarre sense of humor. He relishes cartoons and films such as *E.T.* He also thoroughly enjoys animal programs, and can name a huge variety of animals.

It is good to be able to finish positively. We were desperate when Nicky was deteriorating. No one was able to help, and we had no idea where it would end. Looking back, we can see how much he has improved. Once we let ourselves take advantage of the help that was available, our lives turned around. We also met some wonderful people. Nicky still has a very long way to go. His abilities will undoubtedly always be very limited, and he will need much special help. Like all parents, we want the very best for all of our children. Provided we keep his life simple, predictable, and nonthreatening, Nicky seems to be happy and content. It is these two qualities—happiness and contentment—that we wish for Nicky, above all else.

Postscript

Shortly after the story of Nicky was completed, he started attending Hohepa, a Rudolph Steiner boarding school for disabled children situated on a 70-acre farm close to Napier. It is allied to the Camphill schools and is the only one of its kind in New Zealand.

Although we were very hesitant about Nicky's going away to school and very sad when he eventually went, the decision has proven to be a extremely positive one. During the term time, we are, at last, able to live as a normal family. Meanwhile, Nicky has settled into life at Hohepa well and seems to be happy there. He still has his "ups and downs," but his volatility has continued to decline. Consequently his concentration, though still very limited, is better and he is able to achieve more. We can only put this down to the calm, caring atmosphere created by the extremely dedicated staff and the structured but stimulating routine of the day in this unique community.

Days at Hohepa start to the sound of the flute and finish with a candlelit ceremony. In between, a combination of music, mythology, arts and crafts, drama and eurythmy, and healthy food and exercise, as well as basic reading, writing, and arithmetic, provide a holistic education and life experience. Routine to the year is supplied by the many festivals throughout the different seasons. These festivals enrich the imagination in the way that television, which is not watched at Hohepa, never could.

As for Nicky's increasing achievements, since going to Hohepa, his domestic skills have improved incredibly; he gets great satisfaction from simple jobs like folding clothes, burning rubbish, clearing the table, and generally tidying up. On the school side, he still finds some aspects of the work very threatening—writing, in particular, is a real chore—but he seems to be developing useful skills at craftwork.

Lifestyle choices available for people like Nicky are very limited, and we have investigated all his options. We feel very fortunate that Nicky is able to go to Hohepa. We are very enthusiastic about him being part of such a caring community, with its rich yet accessible culture and unique ideals. As for the future, we hope that Nicky will be able to enter the associated adult community and maybe work in one of the workshops or on the farm.

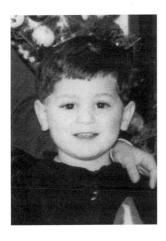

Three

Searching for the Blue Fairy
Thomas's Tale

by Madeline Catalano

Where are you Blue Fairy with your brilliant light?
We need you to rescue us from this plight.
Show us the way to make things right.
Is there a "happily ever after" in sight?

Turn our boy of wood into one who is real,
A boy who can speak, understand, play, and feel.
Research the cause,
prescribe the treatment,
we'll take action,
to achieve satisfaction.

To have our boy "real" again is our dream.
So please send down your luminous beam,
from the far-away wishing star,
and touch him with your magic, wherever you are.

April Fools

I might have surmised that when my third baby "broke the water" on April Fools' Day, 2 weeks before his due date, his life would punctuate ours with many future surprises. Rushing to the hospital, Bob and I joked about telling this unpredictable baby how he had "fooled" his parents at birth.

"It's a boy," bellowed Dr. Leonard. "A boy," echoed Bob, his smile reflecting pride and wonder. The baby cried softly for several seconds as the doctor lifted him. He stopped crying as he was placed on my abdomen. "Do you have hold of him?" asked the doctor. "I've got him," I said, feeling a strange sense of uneasiness as memories of previous strong and persistent newborn cries came back to me. This infant had an angelic face. Compared to his siblings' appearances at birth, his features were perfectly formed.

"This one is good-looking," pronounced Bob. I quickly rationalized the lack of crying as an individual difference. Thoughts of a nonvisible handicap were pushed far aside. The baby was physically healthy, and I had already witnessed normal to outstanding cognitive development in my older children. I basked in the happiness and good fortune of having this beautiful baby boy.

Because of our professions, we were keenly aware of birth defects. Bob is a pediatric ophthalmologist; I am a speech therapist. Both of us have treated children with various disabilities. Only 2 weeks earlier, my best friend adopted at birth a daughter with the rare anomaly of bladder extrophy. This event further fueled my thankfulness for a "physically" perfect child. "He has the best features of both of you," said Dr. Leonard. I agreed and breathed a tremendous sigh of relief as I silently thanked God for the blessing of having three healthy children.

In hindsight, Thomas's lack of a strong cry at birth was the first hint that something was wrong. His reaction to circumcision was the second subtle sign. I watched and winced as three infants screamed in agony during their circumcisions. Then Dr. Leonard entered the nursery to circumcise my baby. "You'll see I have a magic touch," he said. Sure enough, Thomas did not even flinch during the procedure! Dr. Leonard beamed with obvious pride at his expertise. Being naive, I was greatly relieved that this particular doctor had performed my son's circumcision. Two years later when I witnessed my fourth infant's circumcision, there was no such relief for him or me!

Biblically, Thomas means "the twin." In retrospect, this was unfortunately foretelling of his two lives. At 4 years of age, Thomas experienced a regression in emotional, social, and cognitive development that permanently altered his personality. Within the short span of 4 years, Thomas functioned as two different persons. Our first Thomas had no difficulty learning language and social skills. Although his physical appearance was unchanged, our second Thomas behaved "autistic-like." This Thomas's cognitive abilities were impaired, as well as his comprehension of reality and his former self.

Thomas's first 2 years of life were unremarkable. He smiled, attained motor milestones, and said his first words within the range of normal development. Thomas reached out to be held and loved to turn around in my arms and yell out "Bob" when he saw his father. At age 18 months, Thomas toddled about handing family members toys while saying "hall" (*here*). Besides "Bob," by 2 years of age he also said "bye-bye," "uh-oh," "up," "in," "ba" (*ball*), "ca" (*car*), "fly," "ma-ma," and "da-da" appropriately. When asked what sounds certain animals make, he answered correctly. Thomas also pointed to body parts correctly. He pretended to eat toy food by saying "um mum mum," putting the pretend food to his mouth.

Through his third year, my principal concerns about Thomas were that recurrent ear infections would affect language development, and that his expressive language was not as advanced as his older siblings' had been at the same age. I quelled my first worry by recalling that Thomas's sister, Ruth, also endured frequent ear infections, and her language development had been superior. Because Thomas's receptive language appeared age appropriate, I also temporarily laid my second concern to rest.

When Thomas was 25 months old his brother Matthew was born. The day Matthew came home I placed him in an infant seat so that Thomas could see him. Thomas immediately started crying and threw himself face down on the floor. This certainly was a surprising reaction! Bob and I increased our efforts to give Thomas extra attention, believing this to be simple jealousy. However, I could not help but compare this "over reaction" to the milder, more inquisitive reaction of my son Chris when he was presented his newborn sister, also at age 25 months. During Matthew's first 2 years of life, Thomas often tried to hit or push him. I was afraid to leave them alone together. Out of frustration, I told myself, "every child's personality is different" whenever Thomas exhibited unpredictable aggression, as well as tenderness toward his baby brother. I knew that Thomas had the understanding and capability to be gentle. I wished I could trust that Thomas would never harm Matthew, yet a nagging doubt remained.

Delayed Language?

Although Thomas spoke in short sentences at age 3, he did not use personal pronouns other than *I*. His rate of speech was also slow. He had difficulty understanding abstract language and rarely asked questions. His articulation of words was poorer, and his spontaneous speech occurred less often than that of other children his age. These speech/language concerns prompted Bob and I to list Thomas's developmental strengths, to alleviate our mounting anxiety.

We felt that Thomas might be shy and immature, but he certainly was not mentally retarded. He exhibited good receptive language, direction-following, eye contact, and quick learning by imitation. Thomas imitated many things Bob did. He exactly imitated Bob's body postures, even drinking from his own "coffee" cup at the same moment. He wore "potato head" glasses around the house, because his Dad wore glasses. In the morning, Thomas "shaved" with his father using a pretend razor, carefully watching and imitating every move. Thomas also enjoyed "mowing the lawn," pushing his toy mower next to Bob's mower. By age $3\frac{1}{2}$ years, Thomas could expressively identify colors, numbers, letters, shapes, as well as some sight words. He had a long attention span for putting puzzles together, listening to storybooks, and watching *Sesame Street*. His behavior at preschool was socially appropriate. Thomas took toys down from the shelf, played with them, and then put them away as the teacher instructed. Although he expressed little interest in playing with other children, he followed and imitated their play. Thomas especially enjoyed playing "doctor" with his gingerbread man stuffed toy, and with other children. He took turns using the equipment appropriately. He demonstrated imaginary play by building a "house" out of couch cushions and a "Mickey Mouse" out of three pillows. While pretending, he proudly explained what he was doing.

Despite these accomplishments, Thomas also displayed some disturbing negative behaviors. He tantrumed whenever I could not understand what he wanted because of his poor articulation, and his rough handling of his younger brother continued. Little did I know that within a few months, I would have gladly traded these worries for the ones with which we would be faced!

Several rationalizations lessened the gravity of my concerns. Friends consoled me with "Einstein-like" stories of children who were "late" to talk, but eventually surpassed their peers. Disruptive behavior was explained as the "terrible twos," which often extended into 3 years of age. I consulted a pediatrician who assured me that with the start of kindergarten, I would see a surge in Thomas's language development, and a maturing of his behavior. The consensus was that Thomas would "grow out of it." I was willing to take stock in this theory, whatever "it" was!

Fear

Several occurrences between ages 3 and 4 changed these worries to fears. Although impressed by Thomas's letter/number recognition and puzzle performing abilities, the preschool teacher felt that Thomas had a hearing disorder because he did not respond to her calling his name, or initiate speech in the classroom. I had Thomas's hearing tested and the results were normal. It was also unnerving that Matthew was now speaking clearer, using longer sentences than Thomas. Based on my public school experiences, I feared that Thomas would be teased if he exhibited "different" behaviors or was "slow" to learn. I had witnessed the problematic lives of learning-disabled/mentally retarded children made painfully worse by the cruelty of peers and sometimes teachers. Moreover, some teachers fail to meet the challenge of teaching "slow" children; they believe it a waste of their time. An educational supervisor once said to me: "This student has an IQ of 60, why bother, you can't get blood from a turnip." These factors, plus difficulties comprehending "life" in general, could lead to low self-esteem as the child becomes aware of his intellectual inferiority. I was much more worried about Thomas's future mental health and happiness than his intelligence. After all, one's psychological state can compensate for cognitive deficits and often dictates how hard one will work to improve abilities.

Between $3\frac{1}{2}$ and 4 years of age, Thomas displayed many atypical behaviors. Although each was within the range of "normal" development, their sheer number and frequency painted a disturbing picture. Thomas often spun himself in circles. Toileting accidents were more frequent, and he seemed indifferent toward them. He was terrified of vacuum cleaners and public restroom hand dryers. He also cried out in panic when his sleeves became slightly wet while washing his hands. When this occurred, he insisted on taking off all of his clothes, not just the shirt with wet sleeves. He also removed his clothes several times while riding in the car. We had recently moved to a new house and Thomas excessively (or perhaps obsessively) said, "This is Mickey Mouse's house." He displayed repetitive hand-washing and tooth-brushing for 1- to 2-hour periods of time. I recognized these as components of an obsessive-compulsive disorder, but had never heard of this disorder in young children.

Two highly unusual behaviors, however, caused us great alarm. Thomas began awakening in the middle of the night laughing bizarrely. These spells would last for 5–10 minutes, and occur several times per month. I was panic-stricken. The eerie laughter brought to mind long-ago stories of "lunatics chained in the attic" or "insane asylum" characters. In addition, Thomas became obsessed with banging his head on Matthew's head. Only Matthew's head would do! He cried frantically when I restrained him and only after he ran to Matthew and banged heads was he satisfied. This was later replaced by Thomas's biting and then pulling out Matthew's hair (with his teeth), an activity he appropriately called "eating Matthew's hair."

The month before Thomas turned 4 years old (March 1992), he contracted chickenpox. Two weeks later, he began asking "what" and "where" questions for the first time! I was thrilled to hear Thomas say, "I need to go to the bathroom," and then go by himself. He also said, "Come on Matthew, let's go," took Matthew's hand, and led him out of the bathroom. He began to make new observations as indicated in statements such as "Wait a minute, my teacher sings that song!" He even requested a big red ball for his fourth birthday. Bob and I joked that the chickenpox must have improved Thomas's expressive language. Once again we were reassured that he was on the way to overcoming his language delay and catching up with his peers. The week after Thomas's fourth birthday (April 1992), Bob videotaped the children at an Easter egg hunt. Thomas demonstrated good spontaneous speech such as "Here's your basket, Matthew," "Look Daddy, I have 23 eggs in my basket," and "I found it! I found your camera top, Daddy." Little did I realize this videotape would be our last recorded memory of our "normal" Thomas. I could not have imagined that cognitive abilities and mental status could deteriorate so dramatically (given no physical trauma) over such a short period of time.

Nightmare

Grief and terror strike like a bolt of lightning.
We experience a nightmare very frightening.
Some invisible, unknown enemy throws a dart,
piercing our heart, ripping our happiness all apart.
Rendering us helpless, at the mercy of a chaotic disorder;
the sanity of living becomes life on the border.

Awakening we become conscious of our situation,
of which there is no explanation.
Is it easier to deny,
than to ask why?
Do we dare become aware
of an altered reality, which is so rare?
With awakened knowledge comes pain and heartache.
Reality is the nightmare from which we cannot awake.

Breakdown or "Major Developmental Regression"

When Thomas was $3\frac{1}{2}$ years old, he underwent a speech/language evaluation. The evaluation concluded that Thomas would benefit from attending the local rehabilitation center's language-based preschool program. A prerequisite was a psychological assessment, which was administered in March 1992. "Average to above average" results in cognitive and social skills were determined from a battery of tests. One month later, Thomas's cognitive, social, and emotional functioning began to change. Two months later, I made made an appointment with the same psychologist. Obviously shocked by Thomas's new demeanor, the psychologist attempted to conduct a second evaluation using the same tests. He documented in Thomas's second psychological assessment that "clearly, this youngster has experienced a major developmental regression."

When Thomas was exactly 4 years 3 weeks old, he awoke very upset, screaming, "I need to comb my hair!" He combed for several hours with no apparent relief. He continued to cry and repeat this sentence. Although physically present, his dark eyes reflected a mind that was far away and deeply troubled. A terror in his eyes bespoke an internal struggle, as if being tortured by an unseen enemy. That day, I understood the meaning of "tormented soul." Thomas remained distraught all day. He would not calm down or make eye contact. I met Chris and Ruth in their school parking lot that afternoon to try to explain what was happening before they saw Thomas, who was in his car seat in a catatonic-like state. He was staring straight ahead with his eyes wide open and his fists clenched. Although unresponsive, he was producing "growling" sounds. Chris's and Ruth's faces mirrored my own devastation. After months of wondering and sensing that something was drastically wrong with Thomas, we all knew that he had hit rock bottom.

I realized this called for immediate action before Thomas slipped even further away. Nonetheless, I was frozen with shock and disbelief as I helplessly watched Thomas mentally "fall off a cliff" with no safety net in sight. I knew our rapidly descending airplane would most likely crash, but the reality of the situation had not reached a conscious level. Trying to be rational, I could not fathom what insidious, devastating process was occurring. No physical trauma had taken place, yet mentally something had snapped. I wondered where to turn to rescue Thomas from this sudden and severe mental anguish. Although I felt a great sense of urgency, if I rushed him to the emergency room, what would I tell medical professionals? "Please help my 4-year-old. He appears to be losing his mind." What physician would not think something was wrong with a mother to say such things about her own child? After the sudden onset of what has now been diagnosed as Childhood Disintegrative Disorder (CDD), Thomas's behaviors changed daily, and were often bizarre. I was greatly surprised to see that many of his behaviors were the same as those of autistic and psychotic children. This was quite an enigma as my experiences with autism told me it did not just "happen" to a child at 4 years of age! We hoped against hope that Thomas would "snap out of it."

Some of Thomas's problematic behaviors included: destruction of property, aggression toward objects and self (biting his hand and poking his eyes), licking, chewing, or eating nonfood items, obsessively spinning in circles, and climbing high on shelves and furniture. He lost all eye contact and his emotions changed quickly (within seconds) from anger to frantic inconsolable crying, and from silly giggling to fear of ordinary objects! The rapidity of mood swings suggested that a switch in Thomas's brain was being flicked on and off! Amazingly, he remained composed during his school hours (two mornings per week). His facial expression, however, was quite peculiar. He appeared stunned and strained. He seemed to construe that by forcing his eyes to be wide open, he could remain calm and controlled.

Severe agitation made it difficult for Thomas to fall or stay asleep. Sometimes he shook during sleep. Often, he would awake during the night in a hyperactive state. He jumped up and down on the furniture and ran through the house laughing. Some nights he awoke crying in terror, as if having a nightmare from which he could not awaken. These nights it took many piggyback rides from his dad to calm down Thomas.

Thomas also verbalized psychotic ideations. For several weeks, he awoke screaming, "Don't do it to me!" During breakfast, he sometimes yelled, "Don't do it to the oatmeal!" He would frequently cry out, "Take it off," gesturing frantically to his head. His sister Ruth even tried cutting his hair, but that did not reassure Thomas. Several times while pointing to his mouth or nose, he hollered, "Take it out." Other strange sentences, shouted in great distress, included: "There's air in my sneakers!", "There's wind on my face!", and "Don't step on the floor!" These anguished cries demonstrated the helplessness of our circumstances. Thomas was demanding the impossible. There was nothing we could do to alleviate his suffering and rectify this perplexing situation.

Some of Thomas's utterances, as well as behaviors, indicated visual hallucinations. It was with great excitement and interest that he said, "Look Mommy, the stairs are moving" (while he pointed to the stairs), "The drawers are moving" (while he pointed to the dresser), and "The floor is moving!" At times, Thomas appeared to hold conversations (by speaking in gibberish and gesturing) with imaginary people. Frequently he appeared to be seeing something frightening on staircases. He was not only afraid to walk up or down stairs, but when he reached the top his physical posture indicated that he perceived the floor to be "moving."

Some statements were suggestive of "split-personality" or childhood schizophrenia. Several times Thomas said, "Mommy, you have the wrong Thomas," and "Mommy, this is the other Thomas." In June 1992, Thomas said to me, "I don't want to be a different Thomas" (in a desperately upset wailing tone of voice). These words were the most heartwrenching I ever heard.

Thomas's speech, language, and social skills continued to degenerate for 6 months following the onset of CDD. During May and June 1992 his speech became whispered, despite our requests for him to speak loudly. Thomas's talking then ceased. Surprisingly, however, he sang parts of songs every night. He then stopped following directions, and appeared to have lost most receptive as well as expressive language abilities. Further, he stopped assisting in his dressing and toileting. Instead, he physically resisted attempts to dress and toilet him! His behavior appeared disoriented. He would urinate on rugs or on the bathroom door. His confused facial expression suggested he could not comprehend the correct way to toilet himself. Several times, he attempted to drink from toilets as he could no longer ask for a drink. My beautiful once "normal" boy was now acting like an animal; out of this world, in terms of humanness and reality.

The first 2 years of Thomas's disorder were replete with symbolic expressions of frustration, both ours and his. His tearing up of book pages could have represented the ripping of his life into pieces. When he tore off the head of his favorite stuffed toy, "gingerbread man," it was as if his own mind was being ripped apart by internal torment. His knocking over and breaking furniture symbolized the chaotic destruction that replaced our ordinary daily routine. Thomas's pinching and occasional biting of family members epitomized the anger we all were experiencing. His smearing of feces on furniture and carpets (as well as wiping a bloody nose straight across two sets of white drapes) demonstrated the sheer unpleasantness of our altered lives. Why and how did this happen? What was the etiology of this mysterious illness ravaging our son's mind? Was our enemy an inborn genetic brain disorder or an environmental pathogen? Was there a structural anomaly or a metabolic/neurochemical derangement? Had neurological damage been masked by the rapid growth of brain cells during infancy, becoming manifest when brain growth slowed? Was he exposed to chemicals, toxins, or a viral illness? Was Thomas's "breakdown" a manifestation of deep-seated emotional trauma induced by parental pressure to learn, or jealousy of siblings?

While we coped with our guilt, grief, disbelief, and anger, we continued the charade of routine daily living. Our other children deserved some "normalcy" and consistency. No pretenses, however, could change the reality that Thomas was now disturbed and alone in a deteriorating, noncomprehending, and chaotic world. It was as if he was rapidly sinking in quicksand. It was crucial to find the rope so we could pull him out.

Questions and Wishes

What happened to you
my little boy,
so good-looking and sweet,
a real "bundle of joy"?

Everything we hoped for,
a perfect baby to adore.
When did you turn away,
become frightened, refuse to play?
What is causing you to behave this way?
How can we make it go away?

I can tell by your face,
this world has become a scary place.
We love you so much,
please become more in touch.
Why can't you ask "why,"
or even say "hi"?
Be like other children, laugh and play,

look forward to the next day?
Get excited about Santa and the Easter Bunny,
understand why a joke is funny?

We want you to read and write, sing and dance.
Will you have another chance?
You have only one life to live,
we want you to enjoy all we can give.
Please learn to share,
and to care.
Understand dreams, theories and reasons,
appreciate different holidays and seasons.
Learn to swim in a pool,
get good grades in school.

Learn to cook,
have a "favorite" book.
Learn to make a telephone call,
play a game of ball.
Learn to tie your shoe,
be able to say "what's new?"
We hope someday you'll wish upon a star;
look forward to driving a car.
Be "curious," want to learn;
ask brothers and sister for a turn.
Play an instrument like big brother;
relate experiences to father and mother.

You once knew colors, shapes and every letter.
Does this mean you can get better?
Will you ever again pretend,
or make a friend?
We hope your learning will not end.
You can still sing a song,
But can you comprehend right from wrong?
We will always hope and pray
tomorrow you will be better than today.

(I wrote this 3 months after Thomas's "breakdown," while he was still regressing rapidly each day.)

Treatments to Discover on the Road to Recovery

As any parents faced with a child in a crisis would do, after the initial weeks of shock, denial, and depression, we began searching for a cure. Fortunately, our family physician, Dr. Anderson, is extremely competent, as well as compassionate. During our "quest" these past 4 years, he has patiently listened to our concerns, thoroughly researched interventions, and carefully monitored Thomas to determine effectiveness. He guided Thomas through trials of EEG, MRI, and allergy testing, as well as antiyeast and drug interventions.

Dr. Anderson first recommended that Thomas be examined by a pediatric neurologist. Certainly, his distressed and disruptive behavior could be indicative of a neurological disorder. During the 2-month wait for the appointment, I kept meticulous records of Thomas's emotionally labile behaviors, as well as the slipping away of his cognitive and social skills. I anxiously anticipated meeting the pediatric neurologist and assumed she would take great interest in this highly unusual case. Surely, this specialized physician would not only answer my list of questions, but recommend immediate interventions to maximize Thomas's chance of recovery. The appointed day finally arrived. After a 3-hour wait, we were ushered into a small examining room. As the pediatric neurologist briefly checked Thomas's eyes and reflexes, I explained his previously "normal" development, the horrible change that had recently occurred, and our now-desperate situation. In response to my story and list of questions, she shrugged her shoulders and shook her head, appearing totally unconcerned and disbelieving. When I asked if she would recommend an EEG, her response was, "It will do no good." In fact, her only answer to my questions was, "Come back in 6 months and we will see if he is still regressing." I could not believe the lunacy of this "do nothing" advice. Previously, I had thought that the "wait and see" attitude was limited to physicians with little knowledge of neurological disorders. When Bob told her that as a physician himself, given this child's disintegrative condition, he would definitely order an EEG and CAT scan, she reluctantly agreed. Ironically, 2-year-old Matthew suddenly became ill and vomited on the floor. The pediatric neurologist, still expressionless, turned and walked out of the room. When I asked the nurse in the hall whether the doctor would return, she relayed the message that we could schedule our next appointment for 6 months later. We left wondering how the majority of her patients who did not have a physician parent fared. This pediatric neurologist's total lack of interest in the information relating to Thomas's regression, as well as her unfeeling attitude, left us shocked and angry.

We were not about to live with a developmentally regressing, non-sleeping, constantly tantruming child and do nothing for 6 months, only to meet with a repeat performance at our next appointment!

To combat the "I'm all alone in this miserable lifestyle" feeling, and regain the "positive sense" of hopefulness, I read numerous books and journal articles about autistic children. Reading about other parents' difficulties made my troubles seem less in comparison. I was fascinated with stories written by inspirational parents whose searches for effective treatments finally paid off with "happy endings" of greatly improved or "cured" children. These were the treatment ideas to try.

The stories seemed to fall into three categories. The first category attributed autistic behaviors to a variety of physical ailments. When these were eventually identified and properly treated, the "autism" was cured. The second category credited behavioral treatments for autistic children's recoveries. The third category showed physical maturation to be the major factor in dramatically reducing autistic symptoms. Despite behaving quite autistic-like as children, the young adult subjects of these books somehow "grew out of it." In fact, many former "autistics" were able to write their own stories detailing fascinating experiences perceiving the world as autistic children!

One impressive story was that of Jane Rudick's son who was "cured" of Landau–Kleffner syndrome (LKS) by a surgical procedure. I telephoned Jane in June 1992 and was excited to learn that LKS, a rare seizure disorder, closely matched Thomas's regression and late onset of autism. Jane sent me information on LKS, and recommended extensive EEG testing. Although we relentlessly pursued her advice by having Thomas undergo EEG testing in four different hospitals within 2 years, there were no abnormal findings. This was regrettable because obtaining an accurate diagnosis would lead us to effective treatment methods.

Also in June 1992, I began a "magic pill and potion" phase. I noticed that many parents had written letters to autism publications detailing their children's tremendous progress on vitamin, mineral, and/or amino acid formulas. Dr. Rimland's extensive research had shown beneficial results from taking vitamin B_6 and magnesium. Desperately clinging to the hope that a vitamin formula could alter Thomas's "brain chemistry," I crushed and hammered tablets daily for 18 months. I mixed the formula with honey and force-fed the gooey mixture to Thomas who cried and resisted, increasing our emotional stress. Though desperate for Thomas to ingest the "magic potion," I was overwhelmed with guilt at causing a child already ridden with anxiety further distress.

Through further researching the autism literature, I learned that yeast was a major factor in causing an autistic-like condition in several children. This pattern of candida (yeast)-related autism was also connected with antibiotic therapy and contraction of chickenpox at a young age. Again, the description seemed to fit Thomas's disorder. For 4 months, I gave Thomas an anticandida medication and severely restricted his diet. This caused Thomas even greater agitation, as he was obsessed with food. In fact, eating appeared to be his only pleasure during the first year of CDD.

The hope of discovering a rare "cerebral allergy" led me to pursue dietary changes such as systematic elimination of dairy products, eggs, wheat, sugar, fruits, and food additives. I had also read that food allergies could cause hyperactivity, and Thomas certainly had become hyperactive since the onset of CDD. Unfortunately, varying and restricting Thomas's diet effected no change in his activity level, or in his overall condition. "RAST" test results also did not reveal any allergies to foods or environmental agents.

During the first 2 years of CDD, I discovered a "credulity formula." It consisted of a professional's self-confident insistence, mixed with a parent's desperation and naiveté. A physical therapist repeatedly claimed that chewing a large wad of gum would be very "therapeutic" in decreasing Thomas's level of anxiety. Although I knew that this idea was dangerous, as Thomas would attempt to eat the gum and may choke, I allowed her to try. Thomas promptly, with great difficulty, swallowed the large ball of gum. After this experience, I told myself I would certainly never again ignore my own instincts to blindly trust "professionals."

Nonetheless, desperation again led me to a trap offering "cure" as its bait. I took Thomas to an iridologist who had been recommended by several women. Each had credited her with "curing" their cancer. Their faith in this iridologist was so strong that for them she had replaced a medical doctor. Many had their entire families routinely evaluated by her! By looking in the iris of one's eyes, the iridologist claimed she could determine which, and in what way, body organs were ill. To remedy any diseases, allergies, or problem behaviors, she then prescribed "natural" dietary treatments such as herbs, roots, oils, and vitamin supplements. In hindsight, this method seems as reliable as those that determined personality traits by looking at one's body type, or feeling bumps on one's head!

As she looked into Thomas's eyes, the iridologist wrote a long list of "remedies" to be purchased for Thomas to ingest daily. "Keep this list in a safe place. It is your Bible," she said. After insisting that a cure would come from following the prescribed treatment, she announced, "Thomas will be getting some [chiropractic] adjustments!" Then to my surprise she hollered, "Mother, I will check your eyes at no extra charge! Yes, come here. It's all in the eyes. Oh, I see your body is just as full of tension as your son's. Here is a personal program I want you to follow." Against my better judgment, I did purchase some of the "ingredients for a cure" on Thomas's list at the store adjacent to her office. The "extracts" that she said would calm Thomas actually contained a large amount of alcohol. I never did return in 2 months or take Thomas to the chiropractor, as she had recommended. There was too much evidence that her business was not legitimate. The iridologist's name, address, and phone number were not listed in any directory or on her "office" door. She only received clients by "word of mouth" and was supposedly famous as a healer in several countries. I later learned that she worked with the referred chiropractor, and owned the natural foods store where I was to purchase hundreds of dollars worth of prescribed remedies.

One reason I relentlessly pursued physical etiologies was that the alternative would be psychiatric. The old theory that parents, especially mothers, are to blame for psychological problems was still fresh in my mind from college courses. Also, I felt that the stigma of a psychological rather than physical cause would destine Thomas to a life in an institution for the mentally ill. Having witnessed the treatment of patients in several institutions, through experiences as a speech therapist, this thought terrified me.

I read Annabel Stehli's amazing account of her autistic daughter's miraculous improvement following auditory integration training (AIT).

Besides being a noninvasive procedure, the many reported benefits gave me reason for Thomas to try AIT. I learned that AIT consisted of listening to modulated music through headphones for two half-hour sessions per day for a 10-day period.

Improvements in autistic children's functioning credited to AIT include: increased attention span, reduced hyperactivity, improved speech and cognitive skills, and enhanced social appropriateness (including toilet training!). The AIT literature stated that this progress may not be seen for an unspecified period of months following treatment.

It seemed obvious that when children are given many months for teaching, physical growth, and cognitive maturation to occur, the specific effectiveness of AIT may be difficult to measure. Given these additional factors in children's lives, should AIT be given credit for improvements noted 6 months to 2 years following treatment? Despite this intuitiveness, we wanted to try it.

At the onset of our AIT experience, we met many parents who staunchly believed in AIT, as well as in facilitated communication (FC). Several parents had come for their autistic children's second treatments of the 10-day AIT sessions. The woman in charge of administering AIT seemed sincere in her belief that AIT had helped every kind of learning or behavior problem imaginable. She was personable and comforting with a religious demeanor. She emphasized the latter by giving the parents tiny guardian angel pins. Her credentials, which she had previously sent us, were impeccable. They were signed by Guy Berard, the inventor of AIT, who had trained her himself. I was looking forward to her expertise in adjusting frequencies and intensities based on Thomas's reactions to sounds. Frequencies he could not tolerate were to be screened out so his hearing could be "adjusted."

At his first session, I was very disappointed to learn that the only expertise the AIT procedure required was plugging in and turning on the machine (audiokinetron)! I guess I was naive to think that the over $1000 fee per child would entitle each child to attention focused on individual auditory problems. Adding insult, the person administering AIT to Thomas was a college student hired by the woman with extensive credentials and knowledge. After placing the headphones on Thomas, she sat staring at both of us with a bored expression throughout the entire 20 sessions. Hopefully now (3 years later) the audiokinetron may be more easily purchased by organizations so people who wish to obtain AIT can do so for a lower cost. During our 10 days of AIT, many of the other parents expressed their strong faith in FC, which was being hailed as one of the latest "breakthrough" techniques in the autism field. In fact, a psychologist strongly recommended we try FC when Thomas was still nonverbal. At the AIT site, I was interested to see several mothers performing FC with their autistic children using Cannon Communicators. The mother would hold her child's arm so his fingers could press letters to spell words, which were then printed out on a strip of paper. I noticed that the day after the woman in charge announced that our children would be experiencing great stress during AIT because of the change of routine, several children typed out "I feel stressed out" and "I am emotionally upset today." I wondered how seemingly unaware (nonverbal, nonresponsive to directions, self-stimulating) or "low-functioning" children could possess this vocabulary, and type correctly spelled words producing grammatically correct sentences on this little machine, especially with their heads turned away from the letters much of the time! The mothers genuinely believed, and were thrilled, that their children were typing their thoughts.

Several mothers proudly told me that their children were now in age-appropriate grade levels in regular classes at school. Teachers' aides used FC with their children at school enabling them to complete their schoolwork. When I raised doubts that Thomas could spell out and read words, these mothers, as well as the woman in charge of AIT, advised me to "try it." "Your child will surprise you" and "Your child knows so much more than you think he does," they insisted. Their devotion to FC was convincing, and I was tempted, but common sense did not allow dismissal of my numerous doubts. Since then studies have shown that even with the best of intentions facilitators did not realize how much they "influenced" what students typed. Unfortunately, most children could not even type the name of a simple object, unless their facilitators also saw the same object.

During the first year of Thomas's disorder, Dr. Anderson referred us to Dr. Kaye, a child psychiatrist. Dr. Kaye prescribed a small dose of Mellaril, an antipsychotic. This calmed Thomas's destructive behavior, and enabled him to sleep through the night. We will always be grateful to Dr. Kaye for investigating Thomas's unusual disorder and introducing us to Dr. Volkmar. Dr. Volkmar has written extensively about this rare form of autism, which he terms *Childhood Disintegrative Disorder.*

Through Drs. Volkmar and Kaye, we met other families with children with CDD. In February 1994, I began corresponding with Jenny Fairthorne of Australia. Soon after, we began an "international" CDD network. Jenny's wonderful friendship and support have greatly improved my attitude and ability to cope. I was astounded by the similarities of our network members' children. Most notable, with the onset of the disorder each child seemed aware that something terrible was happening to him or her. In every case, this was evident by the child's verbalizations and/or behaviors. Other striking commonalities were sleeping and toileting difficulties, abrupt shifts in mood, hyperactivity, decline in social responsiveness, and difficulty following directions. Language expression and comprehension as well as cognitive skills had regressed, and autistic-like behaviors had developed, in all of the children. The book *When Snow Turns to Rain,* by Craig Schulze, most eloquently describes the feelings and struggles of late-onset autism from a parent's perspective. Jenny and I easily identified with Dr. Schulze's experiences, and have appreciated his insightful input.

Many CDD network members share the perhaps irrational hope that our children have a better prognosis than "typical" autistic children. This hope comes from experiencing our children's promising early development and "normal" functioning. Also, without proof of a structural brain anomaly, a treatable biochemical or metabolic etiology may yet be discovered. When Dr. Kaye recommended that Thomas be seen by Dr. Greenspan, we researched his work. We discovered that he had written extensively on therapy procedures to enable autistic-like children to socially interact with people and their environments. Dr. Greenspan's treatment ideas made sense. He advocated "meaningful" interactive games to playfully force an autistic child to enter into two-way communication. His writings suggested using exaggerated facial expressions and an animated tone of voice, while verbalizing what the child was doing. The goal was to foster "purposeful" rather than "random" activities.

We visited Dr. Greenspan at his home office in Bethesda. After observing us interact with Thomas, he said that Thomas had "islands of communication" that we needed to increase to "continents." He showed us how to "close the circles of communication." As an example, he demonstrated that when Thomas asks to be picked up and we pick him up, we close one circle of communication. We can then expand on Thomas's initiation of interaction by introducing an additional verbalization and action such as asking him if he wants to be thrown up in the air, creating another "circle of communication" to be closed.

Dr. Greenspan also suggested that we imitate Thomas and follow his lead. He demonstrated that when Thomas was purposely playing with objects, we could expand on his play by adding new objects and verbalizations. When Thomas was aimlessly running around a room, we could block his way, without physically restraining him, thereby forcing him to interact with us. To playfully encourage further verbal and physical communication, we could make a game out of the interaction by saying, "You can't escape from me." My favorite suggestion was to actually place significance on haphazard behaviors. For example, if Thomas were to lie on the floor, we could say, "Good night, I see you are going to sleep" and perform bedtime rituals (e.g., give him a blanket, pillow, or storybook). In another example, if Thomas were to spin himself in circles, we could take his hands, turn on music, and say, "You are dancing." Dr. Greenspan said that rather than allowing Thomas to behave in an aimless fashion, we should help him spend more time in a "focused and calm state." This would promote learning, generate spontaneous communication, and hopefully decrease hyperactivity.

Besides Dr. Greenspan's techniques, Dr. Lovaas's method of behavior modification has been most beneficial. This method is aptly described in *Let Me Hear Your Voice,* an inspirational book by Catherine Maurice. I knew from teaching autistic children that once Thomas understood contingencies, he could be taught. My fear was that this comprehension would not occur! Therefore, for the first 6 months of Thomas's regression, I constantly tried to teach Thomas that if he performed a certain behavior (speak, follow a direction, or demonstrate a self-care skill), he would be rewarded with something he desired (food, music, or swinging). This basic principle of behavior modification was the most influential factor in Thomas's beginning to learn skills again. I repeatedly exposed him to language therapy materials, such as picture cards of common objects and actions. I also assembled photograph books of Thomas's interactions with family members and teachers, his performance of chores (during preregression days), and his daily routine. This helped Thomas regain some sense of "self" and "reality" toward his environment.

When eating habits became a problem, several "survival techniques" were implemented. One was placing a combination lock on the refrigerator. This prevented Thomas's habit of constantly opening the door, and consuming any food in sight, including frozen pizzas in their package! Seating Thomas farther away from his siblings at the table discouraged "food grabbing." However, Thomas still had difficulty sitting for meals. He would run around the table, taking food from every plate. Tantrums would ensue when he was stopped. This scene was particularly eerie as Thomas's sister, Ruth, had performed it on stage as Helen Keller in *The Miracle Worker* several months earlier, and only 1 month before Thomas's "breakdown." Eventually, Matthew's highchair was unpacked, and served to isolate Thomas and prevent him from grabbing food.

Self-care skills such as toileting, tooth-brushing, and dressing became very problematic. Thomas developed a fear of toilets, and refused to be near them. In the first year of CDD he became very anxious on entering public restrooms. Instead, he appeared fascinated with "drains" and wanted to urinate into bathtub or shower drains instead of toilets. I took him to the bathroom every 2 hours thinking that a rigid schedule would help "train" him again. Toilets gradually became more familiar, and, therefore, less aversive to him. The number of accidents on floors was also reduced by dressing him in overalls during the day and pajama sleepers zipped up in the back at night. This made it difficult for Thomas to take off his clothes, which he was fond of doing, and "toilet" on a rug or the floor. Presently, Thomas still has difficulty tolerating a toothbrush in his mouth.

A peculiar habit of Thomas's is fingernail biting of his and others' nails. To combat this behavior, I give him baby teething toys to chew instead. In the first year of CDD, Thomas's shirts were turning into "holed cloths" from his habit of chewing small holes in sleeves and collars. To salvage shirts, I cut off the frayed cuffs and shortened the sleeve length making these less accessible for chewing. Thomas made his own "fashion statement," wearing shirts with sleeve lengths just below the elbow, and small holes in the collars. Shirts with buttons could not be worn, as he would bite off, chew up, and swallow small buttons.

The most troublesome aspect of Thomas's CDD is hyperactivity. Directing him to "jump" on a trampoline has been preferable to him jumping on beds and furniture. Even simple structured exercise such as running outside or walking up a hill appears to expend some of Thomas's energy in a positive way, and increases his ability to attend. This is in keeping with the Boston Higashi school, which promotes "exercise" as a main component of their "daily life therapy" for autistic children.

Thomas's hyperactivity would often lead him to run from the house. Installing out-of-reach locks on doors stopped this behavior. The fear of Thomas running into the road, and time spent searching for him outside was eliminated. Another hyperactivity "survival tip" we discovered was the use of a hand-holder or safety strap. (These terms are preferable to *leash*.) This keeps Thomas with me and has tremendously reduced the necessity of chasing him about the house. Teaching sessions and household chores are more efficiently managed when Thomas stays with us, rather than being "on the run." The holder is especially useful in public places such as stores, now that Thomas has outgrown the shopping cart seat. Unfortunately, toileting accidents are more frequent when Thomas is not free to run into the bathroom on his own.

Besides Mellaril, Thomas underwent trials of several other drugs. The first we tried, after discontinuing Mellaril, was naltrexone. He was on this for several months, but we did not observe any changes. Ritalin did not decrease Thomas's hyperactivity, as is reported in children with attention deficit disorder. In fact, Ritalin made Thomas's anxious, upset, and fearful behaviors worse. Prozac and Zoloft have helped reduce Thomas's periods of inconsolable crying, and angry, pinching, and biting behaviors. For Thomas, these drugs have reduced his emotional lability, but have not decreased his hyperactivity.

To date, the best therapy for Thomas appears to be an educational program at home, as well as in school, based on Dr. Lovaas's principles of behavior modification and Dr. Greenspan's methods of social interaction. Emphasis is placed on increasing attention span, communication abilities, and focus of interest on events taking place in his immediate environment. Also helpful is the opportunity to observe and model "normal" behaviors of typical children. Thomas's gradual improvement was not the result of any particular treatment, but rather a combination of approaches. Thomas himself also appears in some way to be adjusting to his new perception of life with CDD.

Keeping a record or diary of Thomas's development since the onset of CDD has enabled us to monitor his 6 months of developmental regression, and note improvements in behavior following this period. A

yearly "behaviors to decrease/behaviors to increase" list has been rewarding to reread as the "behaviors to decrease" have been reduced
from 20 to 6 over these past 4 years.

A Handicap Too Well Hidden

When a mentally handicapped child acts out,
and begins to flail and shout,
their parents receive disapproving glances,
and wide-eyed stares, piercing like lances.
The rude say with their faces,
"I would never allow my child to behave like that in public places."

The already devastated parents are constantly under verbal attack,
"Why can't you control your child?" "He is spoiled and needs a smack."
"That child acts like a fool!"
"Thank goodness he does not attend my child's school!"

A child who acts emotionally disturbed,
causes many to be perturbed.
I wonder why the sight of a physically handicapped child,
elicits reactions more mild.
When people see wheelchairs, comments are not cruel.
Why does a different etiquette rule?

We parents either get angry and shout,
or ignore public reactions, turn away and walk out.
Sometimes we attempt to educate or explain,
to those who adamantly complain.
Other times we casually say, "Good-bye, have a nice day,
my child just happens to behave this way."

We appreciate the rare souls who lend a helping hand,
those who are not quick to judge and reprimand.
Damn those who cause additional complication,
to an already stressful situation.
Parents of children with CDD receive a "bum rap."
"That child looks fine, he can't have a handicap!"
"Normal" appearance is a blessing, from which we cannot win.
CDD is a handicap, too well hidden.

Selling the "Quick Fix" to Parents Desperate to Believe

I can help your son,
the treatmentologist said.
The problem is not just in his head.
His whole body is affected,
it's no wonder he acts rejected.

I am the savior,
I will end his autistic behavior.
Come on my tour
of treatments purported to cure.
I have many for the naive,
those desperate to believe.
They will never conceive,
that I may deceive.
If your belief is great,
my methods will appear top rate.
There is no need to submit to fate,
accept the bait!

After you've searched the medical community,
and paid their exorbitant fee,
why not try a homeopathic remedy?
If you've tried psychology, why not iridology?
Your son is in an unkind bind,
which is upsetting his mind.
He will need chiropractic adjustments,
and many nutritional supplements.

Megavitamins, super Nuthera and DMG,
are readily available for a small fee.
He would be more precocious
if his diet was less atrocious.
Don't be suspicious,
natural foods are delicious.
Eliminate yeast,
restrict his diet at least,
and I'll see,

if he has a food allergy.
And please don't dismiss,
a hair analysis.

Auditory training and sensory integration,
will increase his spontaneous communication.
Try facilitated communication,
experience elation!
You'll be surprised,
to see the genius your son has disguised.
You'll be in ecstasy,
never mind if it's based on fantasy.
And try holding your son tight,
it will eliminate his frustration and fright.

If you cannot change his metabolism,
there is always exorcism!
Perhaps you should focus,
on the theory of hypnosis.
To produce the desired result,
why not try the occult?
In case you have not guessed,
your son is possessed,
with a demon who behaves like a pest.
An incantation I will administer,
to drive away spirits that are sinister.
Or just maybe his particular condition,
will respond to a magician!

The possibilities are immense,
and you won't mind the expense,
once you've become dense,
to reason and common sense.
You need to fix the damage done,
to the innocent victim who is your son.
Yes, there is an abundant supply,
of extraordinary irresistible interventions to try.
Although money-back is not guaranteed,
and some say I am influenced by greed,

there are many for whom my treatments succeed!
Beneficial results are reported by science,
as well as my numerous delighted clients!

My treatments sound illogical and untrue?
What else can you do?
Don't adamantly refuse,
there is nothing to lose!
Given your son's circumstance,
doesn't he deserve every chance?
My credibility is not in question,
I've never had to give a confession.
My methods may seem outrageous,
but the promises I offer are contagious.
As you see I'm most sincere,
so listen to my lure of a cure, without fear.
There are many who applaud,
treatments which may turn out to be fraud.

I would never coax,
or try to hoax!
I promise you will soon discover,
the remedy which will enable your boy to recover!
Now for the tour's conclusion,
I must show you the latest mystical illusion. . .

Hope = Belief + Trust

At the onset of CDD, families experience the grief of losing a loved one. The child's former personality—and indeed his "humanness"—is altered if not lost. Human attributes are replaced by unusual, inappropriate, and often antisocial traits. These changes are extremely difficult to accept when the child's outer appearance remains the same. The first reaction is denial. Then comes overwhelming feelings of shock, guilt, anxiety, and despair. Finally, feelings of acceptance and adjustment are attained. Although parts of these grieving stages will never completely vanish, we eventually can look through the dark clouds, threatening to engulf us, and see the light beyond, illuminating a ray of hope.

Thomas has made slow but steady progress since the onset of his CDD 4 years ago. Instead of a random, nonpurposeful existence, he is now aware of reality and can initiate meaningful interaction with people and objects in his environment. Thomas's increased anticipation of events was recently demonstrated by his spontaneously handing me objects needed to complete actions, such as a camera after being asked "Do you want your picture taken?" and a pizza cutter after he saw a pizza in the oven.

Thomas follows one-step directions and answers many "what," "where," "who," and some "why" questions correctly. He usually responds to "come here" or "come back." In fact, he listened to this command several months ago, just before once again running into the path of a speeding car! Besides the obvious safety benefits, his understanding of directions greatly lessens time wasted chasing him.

Thomas initiates speech for wants and needs. Told to ask for what he wants, Thomas has learned to say, "Can I have?" When upset or frustrated, he spontaneously shouts several unrelated phrases, such as "Thomas says no," "I don't need a bib," "Meow says the cat," and "macaroni and cheese." In the first 2 years of CDD, Thomas would say, "I scared of the dark," as well as "I don't like Mommy" and "Go away Mommy." These phrases greatly increased my guilt and thankfully have completely ceased. Had our experience with CDD occurred during the "refrigerator mother causation of autism" period, I am certain that these utterances would have given validity to this theory!

Thomas's rote memory has also improved. He can recite the days of the week, months of the year, and Pledge of Allegiance. He can also respond to questions about his name, age, birthday, address, and telephone number. Several of his recent requests have demonstrated his ability to remember previous experiences, as well as his increased awareness of reality. One example was his asking for a donut after mass at church and pulling me toward the building where they are available. Another example occurred when he had a stomachache. He asked for and then found the lotion that I had put on his insect bites 4 months earlier. He apparently remembered and generalized the lotion to another situation when he needed to relieve discomfort. This past Christmas, Thomas spontaneously asked for a "ride on the choo-choo train" at the mall. Previous Christmases he had obliviously walked past the toy train ride.

Thomas's speech is sometimes echolalic. At times he appears to use echoing to help him remember correct responses. In unstructured situations, he still speaks to himself in jargon. He sings parts of songs several minutes and sometimes days after hearing them. Unfortunately, his articulation is still poor. He substitutes, omits, and sometimes adds consonants to words, often making it difficult to understand what he is saying.

Fortunately, Thomas's eye contact has improved. It is particularly good when playing interactive games that 2-year-old children enjoy, such as "I'm going to catch/tickle you," "patty-cake," and "this little piggy." His facial expressions show he enjoys these games. He also enjoys looking at books and listening or "dancing" to music. His play skills, attending behavior at school, and fine motor coordination (for tracing letters and "sewing") have also improved. He exhibits appropriate play with toys such as puzzles, balls, blocks, toy cars, and bikes. He can play interactive games, such as rolling a ball back and forth with another person, for several minutes. He recently started to bounce, catch, and throw balls.

Thomas exhibits many of the same auditory processing and comprehension difficulties found in autistic children. He answers questions such as "What color, shape, number, or letter is this?" with responses that, although often incorrect, are always in the correct category. He labels most objects and actions appropriately. However, he still occasionally confuses the names of objects with words that either sound alike (*hamburger* for *hand-holder, dragon* for *giraffe*), are visually similar (*violin* for *broom, carrot* for *pencil*), are categorically similar (*shoelace* for *belt, apple* for *orange, broom* for *mop*), express the object's function (*milk* for *cow, cooker* for *oven*), or are compound words with the first syllable in common (*fireman* for *fireplace, bathtub* for *bathroom, snowball* for *snowflake*). Usually, Thomas can answer questions correctly when given the initial sound of the desired word, the spelling of the word, or the first word of the desired sentence. Reminders to look at the object/action and use of edible reinforcements help to focus his attention and maintain his motivation during therapy sessions. Thomas will delay several seconds before following a direction. He appears to need to repeat the command to himself and process it, before he can carry it out. He responds to directions best with no background noise present. Informal assessment of his hearing shows it to be within normal limits.

When "cookie" is whispered from another room, Thomas will run in to get one!

Thomas also exhibits sensory integration problems typical of autism. He appears to need tactile and deep pressure stimulation, and will seek it out in various ways. He asks to be scratched or brushed, to have a rolling pin rolled on him, and to press his nose against my forehead. Thomas also craves tight hugs, piggyback rides, rolling up in rugs or blankets, and squeezing in between cushions or mattresses. He enjoys lying in tight places such as between the back of a couch and a wall. He also runs his hands over objects, floors, walls, and other people's hands, evidently enjoying the "feel" of textures. Further, he seeks out small holes into which he can place his fingers. On many occasions, we have had to remove his finger from a shower drain, shopping cart slot, and the like. He occasionally licks objects, walls, and pages of books, and frequently chews plastic toys, paper, cardboard puzzles, and household objects.

Thomas always desires food and never appears satiated. Recently, he has begun to yell "yes, yes, yes!" at the sight of food. However, Thomas's obsession with taking food out of the refrigerator has dramatically decreased as has his ingestion of nonfood substances. In addition to food, he thoroughly enjoys chewing his fingernails and toenails. Worse, he now attempts to chew other people's fingernails as well as elbows! Since the onset of his disorder he has had a high pain threshold. He has touched hot objects (e.g., stove, light bulb, fireplace door) and received minor burns, but has not as much as whimpered. When his blood was drawn, he displayed great fear toward the needle and struggled to escape, but there was no indication of pain as the needle penetrated his arm, as he was looking away. Finally, he craves being in high places and literally "climbs the walls." He appears quite agile and adept at balancing on top of swing sets, junglegyms, countertops, and bookshelves. He has occasionally fallen and received bruises, again without apparent discomfort.

Despite being constantly on the run, Thomas is capable of short intervals of sitting while performing academics or watching television. He enjoys jumping from high places onto the floor, jumping on beds, and swinging on doors while standing on the doorknobs. This "off the wall" behavior has literally caused doors as well as curtain rods to come off the wall! Because of this hyperactivity, Thomas needs constant supervision to keep him on task and from running away. This means a "one-on-one aide" at home, at school, and in public places. Besides "watching" Thomas to keep him safe, we have taken extra measures to childproof our house. Apart from locks on outside doors, poisonous or breakable items are out of reach.

Thomas's personality has changed through the course of CDD. At the onset, he resembled "Oscar the Grouch" and "Cookie Monster," obsessed with either breaking or eating. Now he is more a "Curious George the Monkey" character. Property damage is now the result of exploration rather than obsession or aggression. Thomas still chews, disassembles, and/or breaks objects. However, he performs these actions with the curiosity of a toddler rather than with the tremendous anger and frustration he displayed during the first 2 years of CDD.

Interestingly, he has definite storybook preferences, and a sense of humor about characters he finds amusing. Perhaps to reassure himself that he is not alone in his personality, Thomas enjoys characters with which he can identify. He laughs during segments of Sesame Street books where Oscar displays his broken objects and Cookie Monster eats every food in sight, as well as nonedibles. Thomas also laughs during versions of "Goldilocks and the Three Bears" when Goldilocks eats all of baby bear's porridge and breaks his chair. He also enjoys stories and illustrations about animals who chew up household objects. Thomas stares in fascination at an illustration depicting a boy who just hit a ball that broke a car window and the angry car owner. He also spends time looking at illustrations of children making messes or pouring water onto floors, especially when they also depict an annoyed mother. He loves the nonsense segments of Dr. Seuss's books, such as when the Cat in the Hat ate a cake in the bathtub. Finally, he enjoys being read "Curious George" books, as George always gets into mischief.

In a sense, Thomas's enjoyment of viewing mischievous and destructive behavior is shared by his higher-functioning peers and society in general. The success of movies such as *Dennis the Menace, Problem Child,* and *Encino Man* proves that although antisocial behaviors are frowned upon and undesirable to live with, these same autistic-like behaviors are thoroughly enjoyed on the screen by the viewing public!

Although Thomas seems to know that certain behaviors are not socially acceptable, he will still on occasion pull off someone's glasses, rip a book, knock over furniture, cut his own hair, open food items at the store, and put grass or dirt in his mouth. Recently, Thomas has thrown books out of the car window. I receive no pleasure stopping my car on busy streets, and running down sidewalks searching for tossed books, only to find them days later, rain-soaked. Thomas will say "no!" when asked if people should do these things. His facial expression demonstrates some fear of being caught, but also fluctuates between remorse and enjoyment. On the positive side, Thomas's knowledge of his own actions and their consequences represents increased awareness of his environment.

I have found that a sense of humor helps me remain positive. One typical trip to the library entailed Thomas "greeting" a large tank of fish by reaching his hand in to remove them! When the surprised librarian approached, I nonchalantly said, "Oh, he was just saying hello to the fish." It was then necessary to tell Thomas, "We don't eat chairs at the library." Later, the librarian heard me tell Thomas to "stop licking the books" and "stop climbing up the shelves." While absurd scenes such as these are taking place, I cannot help but smile. However, I cannot tell whether this reaction comes from the obvious humor of public reactions to autistic behavior, sheer embarrassment, or some acquired coping strategy. It is more likely the latter, as an attempt at emotional detachment shields me from further psychological pain, after 4 years of bombardment with public disapproval and humiliation.

As Thomas himself has become more accustomed to living with CDD, he has changed from a nonverbal, constantly crying or laughing, noncompliant, disoriented child to one who takes some notice of the world around him. There has been a drastic reduction in mood swings. Emotional outbursts (scared, anxious, and upset behaviors) are infrequent and of shorter duration. Many socially unacceptable behaviors have been eliminated. This year we were thrilled to see Thomas self-initiate toileting and dressing. Thankfully, he currently sleeps through the night, although "bedtime" is around midnight. We know now that Thomas can retain information and is capable of learning much more. Life with CDD is still challenging and difficulties will no doubt continue in the future, but life no longer seems impossible. Although all through our lives we may be compelled to search for the "Blue Fairy," Thomas's progress has given us hope that enables us to face the future more positively!

We Aspire to Inspire

We take actions which keep up hope,
in our confidence and ability to cope.
Even though our child may resist,
we continue to teach and assist.
Of all our resources we take stock,
to try to open the mystery lock.

We enlist expert advice,
no matter the price.
We help him all we can;
we formulate the best plan.
One day we'll find the key,
that will change his destiny.
In the future we will see,
our child happy, healthy and free.

Sibling Thoughts

Having a brother like Thomas may not be easy. We have to watch and care for him much more than a normal child. Although having a brother like Thomas has some positive effects. One good thing is that Thomas has given me a whole new way to look at life. It is easier for me to accept other people's differences and problems. Ruth, Matthew, and I were perfectly normal children. Having a child like Thomas around shows us that having an average family is not something people should take for granted. Another good point is the fact that Thomas bonded our family together. We learned that we all need to work together to achieve the goal of teaching Thomas. If we don't work together, he won't learn anything. Every member of our family, in his or her own way, helps Thomas learn.

—Chris Catalano, age 13

Four years ago, I thought Thomas was fine. He talked, laughed, and played. I never imagined that he would have CDD. I probably would never have heard of CDD if Thomas did not have it. Thomas is one year younger than our cousin, Gina (she used to be our neighbor). Every year, Gina was talking more and more. Every year, I waited for Thomas to talk as well as Gina, but it did not happen.

Thomas is still a very nice boy. I really like him, but some-times he gets on my nerves and I feel like screaming! Sometimes he cries and runs into a closet or bed. Sometimes he can't stop laugh-ing. Sometimes he wants a bunch of piggyback rides. I worry about whether my brother, Thomas, will ever be a normal child. I want Thomas to get better so I can teach him to play baseball with me! I can't automatically make him better by giving him some medicine, but I can do work sessions with him and help him learn. I always will love him.

—*Ruth Catalano, age 11*

I call Thomas my "big, little brother." Sometimes I call him my "hy-peractive brother." When I was 2 years old, I asked Mom, "What's wrong with Thomas?" When I was 3 years old, I asked Mom, "Why does he act like a baby?" When I was 4 years old, I thought he acted like a doggy! Now I help bring Thomas back when he runs away. I help teach Thomas by asking him, "What's this?" and telling him the answer if he doesn't know it. I read books to him. I wrestle with him. I hug him and I kiss him.

—*Matthew Catalano, age 5*

Two Little Boys

Two little boys in the same family.
One as excited by life as can be,
he smiles with anticipation and joy,
when unwrapping a gift or playing with a toy.
For him each day is an adventure to explore,
forever saying, "tell me more."
For him the miracle of life never ceases;
each day his happiness increases.

The second boy, his brother;
perceives the world as another.
Nearly the same age, and in the same family,
he should be sharing life with his brother daily.
Since he developed Childhood Disintegrative Disorder,
his life has become limited, he lives on the border.
For him happiness and participation,
have been replaced by frustration and isolation.

One boy growing up successful and lucky,
making friends to share good times and keep him company.
The other, life did abandon,
anxiety is too often his only companion,
Life will never be able to rationalize,
inequities of enormous size.
Two little boys in the same family,
they lead separate lives as a result of CDD.

Four

Coming Home

by Marie Day

It seems as if it was only yesterday. I remember too well the first incident, the behavior that was so out of character for Aaron. I was vacuuming the living room and he ran across the room and yanked the cord
out of the wall. I was surprised. He had never done that before. I insisted that he plug the vacuum back in. As we fought over control of the
cord, he steadfastly refused, shouting "it's too loud" over and over
again. Losing the battle, he stomped off to his bedroom, and proceeded
to open and slam his door several times.

We repeated the same scene several days later. Worse, he seemed
even more upset. Without explanation, he had suddenly developed
great dispassion toward the vacuum. Considering it a "battle of the
wills," I refused to give in, and continued to vacuum until I was finished. He would either fight for control of the vacuum or retreat to a
floor above or below where I was vacuuming.

Four years old. Pushing his parents to the limit. Testing his bound-
aries. "It's okay," I told myself. "Give it a week and it will all be over."
Only it wasn't. After the next incident, I realized something was not
quite right. From then on, our lives have never been the same.

Aaron was born healthy, and full-term, weighing in at just over 8 pounds. My pregnancy and delivery were uneventful. Through his first 3 months he was colicky and a poor eater. After that he seemed no different to care for than his siblings. He began walking holding onto furniture at 7 months of age, and talking shortly after that. By the time he was 2, his speech was clearer and his vocabulary larger than that of his 15-month-older brother, Cory. Cory was not as outgoing or friendly as Aaron. He always relied on Aaron to take the first step when meeting new playmates. Other parents would often comment on his leadership; he could always manage to convince children, even those a year or two older, to play what he wanted to play.

Aaron continued to learn quickly, make friends easily, and maintain his generous and pleasant personality. He was generally slow to anger, but required no help defending himself. He could blister a foe with a quick and witty response, and his stubborn streak precluded him from ever appearing shy or embarrassed. Generally, however, it appeared Aaron was well-adjusted, had a friendly, outgoing personality, and shared and played well with other children. With regard to health, he had an occasional cold or flu, but nothing more. He was nearly 6 years of age before being prescribed his first antibiotic, for a sore throat.

Several weeks after Aaron's fourth birthday we relocated to a new city. He did not seem upset prior to the move. He was excited and anticipatory. His father and I had promised him a puppy after we moved. He was also moving back to the city where he was born, and where all of his extended family lived.

Only a week after being in our new house did his contempt for the vacuum commence. It was not like Aaron to become agitated over anything, but I also did not consider it truly odd. I was not concerned until a second strange incident occurred. I was in the kitchen when he came in the back door and asked if I would come outside and help him find his "coolit." As I looked around the backyard, I kept querying him: "What is a coolit?" Finally, he ran between the trees and found his water pistol. He began shouting, "I found my coolit!"

"That's a water pistol, Aaron," I said. "You know the right name for it, so why did you call it a coolit?" He never answered me and walked away.

I stood there for a moment watching him. Did he seem a little depressed lately, or was it my imagination? Why did he call his water pistol by another name? At first, I dismissed both thoughts. He was in a new city in a new neighborhood, and maybe "coolit" was the brand name of a new water pistol he had seen on television. I went back inside and completely forgot the event until several hours later. We were sitting with company on our deck. Aaron did not come sit with us or join in the conversation as he normally would have. He stood off in the yard looking up at the sky. Every so often he would run around laughing, and make grabbing motions with his hands as though he was catching butterflies, except there were no butterflies.

Cory had already met a new friend and seemed to be enjoying himself. It was usually Aaron who made friends first. Not only did Aaron show absolutely no interest in joining them, but he became whiny and clinging over the next few days, and began to follow me around the house from room to room. I could not be out of his sight for more than a few seconds, or he would call me in a panic. It began to wear on my nerves, and he refused to answer me when I questioned what was the matter. Then he began to sit on the couch for hours at a time and stare off into space. "No," he did not want the television on. "No," he did not want to go outside. "No," he did not want to play with any toys. When anyone asked what was the matter, he would only answer, "nothing."

My husband, Adam, also noticed Aaron was not himself, but told me to give him some time to adjust to the new environment, and Aaron would be in the swing of things before long. His explanation was that Aaron did not know any kids yet and did not know his way around the neighborhood. In time, he would be as outgoing as he was before. I listened, but by now I did not believe a word of it. Aaron was not showing any signs that he was physically ill, so I dismissed taking him to a doctor.

Aaron's older sisters also noticed that Aaron seemed depressed lately. They decided now was the time for him to get his new puppy, even though he had not mentioned it lately. They drove off and returned several hours later with a tiny 6-week-old male black Labrador retriever. They called Aaron to the kitchen to show him his new puppy. Not only did Aaron show very little interest, at times he acted terribly afraid. He refused to pet the puppy and wandered out of the room. All of us looked at each other, but no one verbalized what was on all of our minds. Physical symptoms or not, it was time to get a physician's opinion. Adam finally realized something was wrong, and offered to consult a doctor the following day. Adam explained to our practitioner that Aaron's personality was changing, that he was becoming very upset over trivial matters, and that he usually failed to respond when he was told to do something. The doctor summed it up neatly. He told Adam that Aaron simply had a behavioral problem that a little firmer discipline would straighten out. Naturally, we knew the doctor was wrong, and did not even consider his advice.

Over the next few weeks, Aaron's behavior changed rapidly and dramatically. Changing from sitting in a stupor and staring into space, he became hyperactive and at the same time fearful. Turning off and on the lights soared into an obsession. Bathing was a task to be abhorred. Even the sound of the bathwater sent him running. Adam would bring him kicking and screaming into the bathroom; we would both have to hold him in the tub. Aaron seemed to have abnormal strength for his age and size. Even with both of us holding, we still could not manage to sit him down. He stood and fought the entire time. That was easy, washing his hair was the real challenge. I decided washing it in the kitchen sink would be easier. With his father pinning him on the counter, I washed his hair. Aaron fought so much that I am certain that for an entire year I was unable to completely rinse his hair of shampoo.

Over the course of several weeks, Aaron's speech became very slurred, and he began omitting parts of words. Juice became "duce," and he sometimes substituted his own made-up word for a common word. He refused to wear certain clothes, and if I fought him into them, he would take them off and run around the house naked. Food he had loved before he refused to eat. If he would eat at all, it would only be something he chose, something either very salty or very sweet. Temper tantrums, aggressive behavior, and destructiveness became a common occurrence. He retreated more and more into his own world. He refused to play with toys or watch television. I was desperate to determine what was happening to him, and would often plead with him to tell me what he was thinking. During these times he always spoke about seeing people in the house, how he heard them talking, and how afraid of them he was. It was very fortunate for Aaron that he was able to verbally express some of what he was experiencing during his regression, as this became helpful in his later treatment. He spoke less and less each day and what speech he still had was becoming increasingly difficult to understand.

Day by day Aaron's behavior became more bizarre. He began holding up his hands and staring at them for minutes at a time, countless times a day. He started shaking his head quickly from side to side, and laughing or crying for no apparent reason. Certain noises would particularly set him off. Every time the phone rang he would jump up in a panic and run around in circles. Of all the changes taking place, the most difficult for me to accept was his loss of toileting skills. The first few times it happened, I always managed to convince myself that it was just an accident and would not happen again, even though it first began during the daytime, while he was awake and walking around. Then it began happening at night, and soon he was barely ever using the bathroom on his own. We would take him and try to place him on the toilet many times a day, but he fought us constantly. It was a losing battle.

I remember clearly the day I decided to put him back into diapers. I went into his bedroom in the morning only to find all of his bedclothes soaked again. By now this was a regular occurrence, not only in the mornings, but just about any time he laid on his bed. I grabbed a corner of the bedding to pull it off, and suddenly I did not feel the energy to change his bed again. I was so tired of changing sheets, sometimes five times a day. I sat on a dry corner of his bed unable to move, and recalled an event that happened approximately a year earlier. Adam, I, and the children were on our way home from buying groceries, and we passed a yard sale. I noticed a piece of furniture that I was interested in, so we stopped to inquire. The people running the sale told us the lady across the street owned it, pointed out her house, and asked that we check with her regarding the price. We knocked on her door and after waiting a minute or two, she answered. We very briefly discussed the piece of furniture and the price she wanted, but she very quickly changed the subject and began reciting a lengthy story about her grandson. She told us that she was his legal guardian, because he was mentally retarded and his mother could not cope with him. As I was digging into my purse for my wallet, the smell of urine drifted past my nose. We made our exit as quickly and politely as we could. After returning to our car, I commented to Adam that just because her grandson was retarded, you would think she would keep the house clean and change his clothes and bedding so the smell of urine would not be noticeable. Sitting on the edge of Aaron's bed, I realized my callousness. That woman had been dealing with her grandson for years; I was burned out after a month. I regretted that I never took the extra time to listen to her. If everyone could walk in another person's shoes for a while, I'm sure the world would be a much more compassionate place.

Deciding to put Aaron back into diapers was one of the most distressing things I ever had to do. It was my final admission that Aaron was gone. We had moved to another city but had taken the wrong child. Even physically, he did not resemble Aaron. His facial expressions were different, his walk was wrong, and his once sparkling blue eyes were now blank. He had the look of the dead. Someone had come and snatched the very soul from his body. All we were left with was his shell.

Aaron's pediatrician had him admitted to the hospital in our city, and consulted a psychiatrist and a neurologist. Extensive blood and urine tests were conducted, as well as a CT scan and an EEG. All test results were normal. Notably, Aaron either showed extreme fear when anyone approached him, or he did not acknowledge their presence at all. The psychiatrist stated he seemed autistic in many ways, but not all. He thought Aaron may possibly have temporal lobe epilepsy. The neurologist thought possibly a leukodystrophy, although Aaron did not have any signs of a neurological problem. The pediatrician was at a total loss. She said that in her 30 years of practice, she had come across only one case very early in her career where "a child lost all his acquired skills, and eventually that child curled up and died." That did not make my day. The doctors decided to send Aaron to a hospital several hours away for an MRI examination.

Three days later, Aaron was in another hospital under the care of a pediatric neurologist who was reputed to be an expert in his field. I became increasingly disappointed as I watched him test Aaron. His examination consisted of taking several little rubber "Bert and Ernie" toys from his black bag, sticking them on his fingers, and waving them around while asking Aaron, who was completely mute by that time, questions that he was totally incapable of answering. The neurologist then ordered more tests, which also included an MRI, and said his blood work would be sent to Boston for complete analysis. We were told that some of the test results would take a few weeks, but we knew fairly soon after the MRI and EEG tests were done that the results were completely normal. It was not a surprise when the neurologist said that so far, he could not find a reason for Aaron's regression.

Several weeks later, I officially heard from the hospital that nothing abnormal was discovered on of any Aaron's tests. The entire process seemed like such a waste of time. I knew it had to be done, but at the same time, I felt guilty putting Aaron through all of this. He had to be sedated for even the most minor of tests. At the time, I thought it would be well worth it, because at the end we would finally know what was wrong with Aaron and he could be "cured" or at the very least, helped. I was very depressed. The doctors were basically saying he was all right—no brain tumors, no rare form of epilepsy, no infection, no anything. It made me want to scream. I had a perfectly normal, happy child only a few weeks ago, and now I had a child who pooped in his pants and stared at his hands. People did not empathize that I could accept Aaron's condition better if he had stepped onto the road and got hit by a car. At least then there would be a reason for the way he was. We would be able to see and know where the problem was. This way, it all seemed so senseless. What a waste of a life.

I thought Aaron's behavior was as bad as it was going to get. What else was left that he could possibly do? He was already completely mute, and extremely hyperactive. He wandered the halls at night, was back into diapers, was aggressive and destructive, and lived in his own world. How wrong I was. He came tiptoeing out of the living room one day hitting himself on the side of his head. He began walking in a sideways, skipping sort of way, and began yelling an irritating high-pitched, "eeeeeeeeeeeh" sound that always ended with a few shakes of his head. He also became obsessed with the face cloth. He would wipe his face and hands in a quick manner, put the face cloth back on the counter, walk a few steps away, turn around, and repeat the process over again. This went on for hours at a time. Sometimes he would take a break from this and stare at his hands, continuing this obsession even while walking or he would walk to the back door, look out, and walk back to the counter and start the face cloth repertoire over again. He also became obsessed with the toaster. He would approach the toaster, look at it, take a few steps away, and then turn around and go back to the toaster. He was in motion constantly, and continually ran around and around the kitchen table. On most days he was afraid to go outside, but on occasion would wander out to the backyard. He smashed all of the yard lights one day, and was particularly fascinated with clothes hanging on the line. He would pull them all off and stomp on them. Our dog, who was no longer tiny, seemed to know Aaron was the weak one in the pack. As soon as Aaron stepped out the door, the dog would bite his pants or grab onto his shirt and hop along on his back legs with every step Aaron took. Aaron would walk across the entire yard oblivious that he had a dog attached to him. I became fed up with all of the torn clothes and decided the dog had to go. Aaron never even missed him.

It became impossible to take Aaron anywhere, especially to stores. He ran around in a frenzy knocking everything off the shelves. Adam said Aaron reminded him of a brush fire in the wind. We were never sure if we should stop and try to clean the mess he already made, or catch him to try to prevent him from doing more. Things got even worse if we managed to make it as far as the checkout counter. Unbelievably quick, he would run to the register and press the buttons, and not just the counter we were at. He would sometimes get to three or four other ones before we could grab him. He had the advantage of running beneath the bars separating the checkout counters, and some people were upset they had to wait for the cashier to correct their total. I am certain most people thought we were raising an undisciplined, spoiled brat. God bless those other people who looked at it with a bit of humor.

What bothered me more was Aaron's unprovoked attacks on strangers. He would run to anyone he picked out of a crowd, either man, woman, or child, and hit him or her. I was always thankful he never hit a baby or toddler, my biggest fear. At 4 years of age, he was still small enough to put in a shopping cart, but sometimes he would create a worse scene if he wanted to get out. He especially liked grocery stores. He would take the apples and oranges and throw them at people or toss them down the aisles. He would squeeze soft food between both hands, and throw bags of potato chips on the floor and stomp on them. We decided to stop taking him into any kind of store.

Approximately 12 weeks after the onset of Aaron's regression, we received his diagnosis of Childhood Disintegrative Disorder. Aaron had lost all of his acquired skills in a matter of only 7 weeks. He had been seeing a psychiatrist every week since his release from the hospital. The day I learned his diagnosis, there were two psychiatrists in the office. They told me that they both concurred with the diagnosis of Heller's syndrome. Aaron fit the full criteria for it, and all of his medical tests had ruled out anything organic as being the cause of his regression. I remember asking a few questions, but even as we were talking I decided

I'd go down to the library that night and get as much information on it as I could. I knew I could get more information at the library than I could get out of the two psychiatrists. "What's the name of it again?" I asked before I left. "Heller's syndrome," his doctor replied. "Heller's syndrome," I thought to myself. "Yeah, life has been hell lately. Easy enough to remember." I left their office happy. "They finally know what's wrong with Aaron. Now they can fix him."

"Usually the loss of skills reaches a plateau, after which some limited improvement may occur, although improvement is rarely marked." That statement haunted my every waking hour, and sleepless hours during the night. Everything I read repeated the same statement. Case histories reported most of the kids were placed in mental institutions because they failed to regain enough skills, and were too uncontrollable to remain at home with their families. One report I read stated that one boy had finally learned to eat with a spoon again after his caregiver had spent 8 years showing him how. Words cannot even begin to describe how I felt. This was the blackest period of my life. Some days I would sit down and my body and mind prevented me from getting up again. I somehow managed to get through the days, look after the kids and the house, and appear all right to everyone who saw me, but I was not all right. What was to become of Aaron? Would he also end up in an institution somewhere? I hated to think about that, but could also see how it could be possible. I felt overwhelmed looking after him for only a few months, and he was still only 4 years old. What would he be like at 15, or even 10? He seemed so abnormally strong at age 4, what would he be like even a few years from now? Every year that passed, I would be getting older and weaker, and he would be getting bigger and stronger.

His psychiatrist insisted on psychological testing. The results placed Aaron between 15 and 18 months of age intellectually. His expressive and receptive language was at the same level. The report stated he used mainly peripheral vision during the interview and his speech consisted mainly of grunts. This only confirmed what I already knew. During one visit to Aaron's psychiatrist, I made a statement in reference to having a child with the mind of a toddler in the body of a 4-year-old. To my further dismay, the psychiatrist suggested I was overrating Aaron. He commented, "No, Aaron is much worse than a toddler. At least a toddler would respond when you spoke to him, but Aaron doesn't even do that." "Great," I thought, "he really knows how to lift a person's spirit."

On another occasion, he told me to accept that Aaron will never be normal again, will always be classified as a special needs child, and will never be able to function in society. I knew he was right. He knew I was trying to hang onto something that was long gone. He also knew I was in denial and refused to accept Aaron's diagnosis. It was 2 years after Aaron was officially diagnosed that I even told our closest relatives exactly what he was diagnosed with. At the time I told friends and relatives that "they think Aaron may have CDD, but the doctors still are not sure. They do not have a firm diagnosis yet." Yes, I was in denial.

Things got worse as every month passed and Aaron would develop another strange habit. He began sticking things in his mouth. He would take a drinking straw or his toothbrush and ram it down his throat until he gagged. He also started carrying strange objects around in his hand day and night. First it was a tiny ball, then a plastic tab that keeps a bread bag closed, and next a tiny plastic gun that was less than a half-inch long. If he managed to displace it for a minute, or if he lost it in the middle of the night, there was no peace until we found it. There were many nights where both Adam and I were in his bedroom looking through his bedclothes, under the bed, and through the carpet. Aaron lost his little gun in the grass one day; it was a miracle we ever found it.

Four months after the onset of Aaron's illness, his hyperactivity and other behavior were exasperating me. He was all I ever thought about. I read everything I could find on diseases that could cause regression in children, and tried to find something in every syndrome that could fit Aaron. Nothing seemed to match. It was either ruled out because he had already been tested for it, or he was the wrong sex, or he was of the wrong ethnic background. I had kept a journal on Aaron that I wrote in on a daily basis. I reread all of my notes. Without a doubt, before Aaron lost his speech entirely, he spoke of things that made me think he was seeing and hearing things that were not there. He was hallucinating. I read over all of the information I had on CDD, or Disintegrative Psychosis, as it was also referred to. It was obvious that someone in the past noticed these children had some form of psychosis before they regressed, as "psychosis" was included in the description of the disorder. For the first time, things were finally making sense.

At Aaron's next appointment with his psychiatrist, I insisted he be prescribed an antipsychotic medication. His doctor refused, and prescribed clonidine instead. I was upset, but agreed to try clonidine, for a while anyway. It did seem to help in the beginning, but after a few weeks, made Aaron white as a ghost, and he would fall asleep for hours during the day. It gave me a break from him, but I knew it would not help him in the long run. In fact, Aaron was still becoming worse, and his behavior more bizarre. He began rolling his eyes upward and poking his fingers into the corners of his eyes. To watch this gave me "the creeps." Then he began spitting. He would spit on the floor in every room he went into, or else he would spit into his hands and smear it on the television screen or coffee table. I failed to understand how he managed to come up with new and strange behaviors on an almost daily basis. I do not think someone faking mental illness could dream up such bizarre behavior but to Aaron, they came too naturally.

Adam and I disagreed, sometimes bitterly, on how to deal with Aaron's aggressive, destructive behavior. We each had our own opinion on how he should be handled. Adam would physically restrain Aaron by wrapping his arms around him. I strongly opposed this method of control. I found it made Aaron even more aggressive, and the episode would last longer. I let Aaron attack the furniture or whatever he was after, as long as it was not another person. I found this worked well for, in a short period of time, Aaron would calm down. Adam disagreed, saying Aaron should not be allowed to get away with unacceptable behavior and should be restrained. However, as long as I was around when Aaron was out of control, I got my way. One day while I was in another room, I heard chaos and knew Aaron was out of control. I walked into the kitchen to find Adam trying to restrain Aaron in his usual manner, and even before I could get it out of my mouth for him to let Aaron go, I was horrified to see Aaron bite himself on the wrist. Self-mutilation. I had read about that. I think it shocked Adam as much as it did me. He promised he would never use the holding method again, and he never has. That was the first and last time Aaron ever bit himself.

At Aaron's next appointment with his psychiatrist, I was determined not to leave without a prescription for an antipsychotic medication, even if I had to chain myself to his desk to get one. When I brought up the subject, I was told that an antipsychotic medication would probably not benefit Aaron in any way, and that the medication has severe side effects. I said I did not care because he does not have a life anyway. The doctor finally wrote out a prescription for an antipsychotic medication, Largactil.

After exactly 18 days, I noticed an improvement in Aaron. Before starting Largactil, he had advanced slightly in some areas, such as playing with an odd toy or two, and he seemed to be less destructive. He would sometimes take our hands and lead us to the bathroom to indicate he wanted to go. He had also begun eating a larger variety of food, and had lost his fascination with the face cloth. These improvements, though, were very slow in coming, and did not seem to go much further until Aaron began taking Largactil. On the medication, he began going to the bathroom on his own and sleeping through the night. His appetite improved, and he had a wider interest in toys and in his surroundings. Until then, he refused to eat or even sit at the dinner table with the rest of the family. Most of the time, he would be off in a different room by himself. This had been another area in which Adam and I disagreed. Adam thought Aaron should be forced to sit at the table with the rest of the family, but I disagreed. To me, it was pointless. Aaron would not eat if anyone was around, and the rest of the family never got to eat either because we were too busy trying to get Aaron to stay in his chair. I would leave a variety of nonperishable food on the kitchen table and Aaron would sneak in when nobody was around and eat.

To the horror of autism experts, I did many things I suppose they would consider sins. Because Aaron withdrew suddenly into his own world, I reasoned he needed to be by himself. I never forced him to be in the company of others, if he didn't want this. I never forced him to go outside, or do anything unless it was of his own choosing. Instead of making the house a stimulating environment, I made things as quiet and as peaceful as possible. I was new at this and figured I would give Aaron the time he needed until he was ready to rejoin the world. That finally happened the night he walked into the dining room, sat down with us, and ate dinner. He seemed nervous and jittery, but managed to stay at least a good 6 or 7 minutes before he was gone again. The next day he heard the mailman come. He went outside and got the mail and brought it to me. It became easier to dress him in different clothes and he actually stayed dressed. He was dry day and night and I was able to pack away the diapers. When he awoke in the morning, he would get up, come downstairs on his own, and eat breakfast at the kitchen table, pointing to the cereal he wanted to eat that day. He would go to the refrigerator and point to either the milk or juice, or whatever he wanted to drink. He stopped spitting on the floor and carrying around a little object in his hand. His eye contact was increasing daily. Things were going well and everyone close to him could see the progress Aaron was making. In another month, Aaron had lost all he had regained, and we were back at square one.

Approximately 6 or 7 weeks after Aaron was on Largactil, even his psychiatrist noticed the change. He commented on how much calmer Aaron was, and how he seemed to even be aware of our conversation. Before, Aaron refused to sit still in the office. He would run around getting into trouble, or would sit on the window sill, banging his feet against the heat register. The noise would echo throughout the building. But this day he sat quietly in the chair next to me, drinking the small container of apple juice I always brought for him when he visited the doctor. After he finished his juice, Aaron calmly walked to the window and stood there for a while viewing the sights. His doctor was not certain if the improvement in Aaron was simply him getting better on his own, or related to the medication. I told him that I was sure it was because of the medication, but he convinced me to take Aaron off the medication on a trial basis. Things appeared all right with Aaron over the following week, but after that, he slowly declined. He began spending more and more time by himself, became very aggressive and hyperactive, and, most depressing, he was back in diapers again. Three weeks later, I started giving him Largactil again. I waited for improvements. After 21 days, Aaron started improving again. Over the course of the next 4 or 5 months, Aaron made remarkable gains. To me, there was no disputing the fact that the medication was helping him tremendously. He began talking again, first using only one word at a time in a very infantile way. He would ask for "milky" or "juicy." He wanted his "mitties" or "sockies." He was completely toilet trained, and we were able to take him into stores again. He was playing with toys and even his brother. He became more sociable and would run to answer the door when the doorbell rang. It was his job to get the mail daily, and he would put his toys away when he was told it was bedtime. Some of his skills were lost for the third time when his psychiatrist decided to place him on a newer and "safer" antipsychotic medication, Risperidal.

Aaron was slowly weaned off Largactil and introduced to Risperidal. He was only on Risperidal for about 3 weeks when I insisted he be taken off that and placed back on Largactil. He seemed to lose some of his newly acquired skills on Risperidal, and it made him nervous and tense. It also made him urinate at least 60 times a day. He began to spend his entire day in the bathroom. After restarting Largactil, it took several months before he was even close to where he was before.

By now, Aaron had just turned 5 years of age. Eleven months had passed since the onset of his regression. He was improving slowly in all areas, but he was still far from normal. Even though only 2 months was left of the school year, we enrolled him in an integrated preschool program. He was aggressive on a few occasions, at which times I would take him home. For the most part, he did not mingle with the other kids, and usually he would refuse to paint or get involved with classroom activities. At times, he even refused to leave the school to play outside. The only thing that was not a problem was taking him to school. He willingly walked into the classroom on his own. Aaron's developmental assessment done at that time placed him between 39 and 42 months of age, with a continued delay in his expressive language. He was still 2 years behind where he should be, but 1 year earlier he was at a 15-month age level. I was optimistic that he was at least advancing. Over the summer, we continued to notice positive results in Aaron. Noise did not seem to bother him as it did before, and he began to ride his bike and take short walks by himself. His speech was now more appropriate. When he first began talking again, there was much echolalia, but he never did reverse his pronouns. When I would ask him if he wanted a cookie, he would answer "Aaron doesn't want a cookie," or when he fell and hurt himself, he would come running saying, "Me hurt me." When I would ask a general question like "Does anyone want more cake?" he would always answer, "Aaron wants more cake." He finally stopped speaking like that. By the summer holidays, things were going well, for the most part. Nonetheless, he still had occasional explosive temper tantrums, and his thinking was still impaired when it came to many things. He appeared to not comprehend certain commands or statements, and much of the time he still seemed to me to be depressed. One outstanding gain he made was the return of a social smile. I had not seen this for over a year. This milestone was one of the most important things that assured me he was coming back. He would smile appropriately, not in some crazed manner over nothing, as he used to.

Aaron began kindergarten in the fall of 1995. I had asked the school board for an aide to help Aaron. His preschool teacher said she would like to see how he managed in kindergarten without one, and her recommendation was that he be given the opportunity to try it on his own. I was dubious, but I did not have a say. Aaron wanted me to walk him into his classroom the first week, and to the back door of the school for the next 2 months. For the next 3 months, I was able to walk him to the back of the school and leave before the bell rang, and for the next 2 months following that, I could drop him off at the front of the school and leave, allowing him 10 minutes or so to play with the other children before school began. By the end of April, he began to walk the four blocks to school and back home again by himself. There was one busy street on which he had to be extra careful, and three streets that were much less busy. I started with the intention of having him walk with his brother, but on the very first day, Aaron came home by himself at noon. He said he did not see Cory when the bell rang, and he did not want to wait for him, so he left without him. I tried not to show my worry, but I was horrified. The same thing happened the next day, and continued throughout the remainder of the school year. On days when Cory was sick, Aaron made the trip by himself both ways and never showed any concern. I considered this a big step in Aaron's independence.

Unfortunately, things did not go that smoothly in the classroom. There were times when Aaron became aggressive and did not comply with his teacher's instructions. Thankfully, Aaron's teacher was patient and understanding and she usually had enough insight to settle matters. There were only a handful of times that I had to go to the school to get Aaron. For the first three quarters of the school year, Aaron seemed to fit in with the other children socially and academically better than I had anticipated, but by the last few months, it was evident that Aaron was slipping behind in both areas. Whereas other children could now print their name with ease and recognize and print other small words, Aaron was still struggling with printing his name correctly. If his teacher stood over him and told him exactly what to do on every step of a worksheet, he could do it reasonably well, but left on his own, he was completely unable to do even the easiest task correctly. His teacher also noticed that while the rest of the children could understand a joke, jokes were beyond Aaron's comprehension. The other kids had developed abstract thought processing. Aaron was stuck in concrete thinking.

By the spring of 1996, I was neither convinced nor did I accept the fact that Aaron had CDD. I was still looking for the "correct" diagnosis.

After another EEG test, his fourth in 1½ years, I convinced his doctor to put him on a trial of an anticonvulsant medication. He prescribed Tegretol. Aaron had to undergo his most feared procedure first, a blood test. I always felt awful when Aaron had to have a needle, or a test of any kind; Adam usually took him. After only 3 days on Tegretol, Aaron started to vomit and broke out in a bright red rash. It was obvious he was allergic to it. That incident finally caused me to wake up and do some soul-searching.

Aaron had already been carrying the diagnosis of CDD for 21 months, but I would not or could not accept it. I requested and was granted referrals to other doctors for other opinions, but their opinions were the same. He fit the profile for CDD. My argument was that maybe he was schizophrenic. Aaron had odd behavior; schizophrenics have odd behavior. Aaron talked as though he were hallucinating before he became mute; schizophrenics hallucinate. Aaron was on an antipsychotic medication and it was helping him. Finally, many schizophrenics lead normal, productive lives. That was what I wanted for Aaron. I wanted him to have a different diagnosis so he could have a chance at life. At least there was hope if he was schizophrenic. From all I had read on CDD, there was no hope.

Aaron's allergic reaction to Tegretol finally made me think about my constant search for another diagnosis. For whose benefit was I putting him through extra tests and sickness? To this day, I am confident that I did it for Aaron, and I do not regret my search for another diagnosis. I know my persistence sometimes made doctors take extra steps to rule out anything questionable. I realized, though, it was time to stop. I had come to the end of the road. The psychiatrist asked me at our next visit, when I was arguing about the possibility of another diagnosis, if I thoroughly and completely understood the criteria in diagnosing CDD. Quickly, I answered, "Yes, of course." "Good," he said, "and do the criteria fit Aaron?" I stared at him. I honestly could not open my mouth. I felt like I stared into his dark eyes for hours, but I know it was probably less than a minute. "Yes," I answered. He gave a slight nod of his head, and that was the end of our argument. I did not expect his question, nor did I expect my answer. After nearly 2 years, he had finally made me face the devil. I felt emotionally drained after leaving. It had finally dawned on me to stop chasing shadows, and start helping Aaron. Smart man.

Two weeks before the end of kindergarten, psychological tests were repeated to determine Aaron's requirements for grade one. By now, it was obvious he would need extra help, at least academically. I could not understand why they would even bother testing him again. His kindergarten teacher showed the psychologist samples of the work Aaron did when left unattended. It was far from what it should have been. Aaron liked to draw windows, and in every space on the worksheets where a word should go, he drew a window. Even a normal 6-year-old could look at Aaron's work and know he needed help, but no, it had to be determined by someone 30 years older, who could use larger words. Lo and behold, the psychologist, according to her testing, which is in her words "always accurate," stated Aaron's IQ was over 70, and out of the "mentally retarded range." Good news in one regard, but not another. According to our school's guidelines, any child who is not "mentally retarded" is not eligible for special assistance. Aaron would be on his own for first grade. I could easily help him academically, but he does not seem to have the patience or concentration to sit with me for any length of time. We both become frustrated. He seems to have a selective attention span. He can play computer games for an hour at a time and devote attention and concentration well enough so that he can win a few games or surpass his last score. Trying to get him involved with something that he has no interest in, however, is nearly impossible.

Aside from his obvious learning problem, Aaron has made remarkable strides forward. He has regained much more than the doctors predicted he would 2 years ago, and they are still surprised that he is continuing to make slow gains. As I stated earlier, he walks back and forth to school on his own. He argues with his brother, calls on a friend who lives around the block, rides his bike, draws and colors, plays games on the computer, does a few household chores, and takes our new dog for a walk by himself. During the school year, he was even invited to several classmates' birthday parties. When I questioned the children's mothers later, they said that they were totally unaware that Aaron had any problems. They perceived no difference in Aaron from the rest of the children. That was very nice to hear.

Is Aaron like he was before? No. He is not the same child I had before. He has made great accomplishments over the past 2 years socially and in life skills, but he is not home yet. I feel he is on his way, and I desperately hope he makes it, but only time will be able to tell us that.

Everyone has their own opinion as to why Aaron has come as far as he has. The doctors think it is part mystery, medication, and Aaron's own doing. Most friends and relatives are of the opinion that Aaron is getting better by himself, without help from anything, and his grandmother thinks it is because he has had so many prayers said on his behalf. A person in the mental health field told me that Aaron had improved because I had the knowledge and ability to deal with him, and I deserved much of the credit. This statement is absolutely false. I know why Aaron improved. Without a doubt, it is because of his medication. The only credit I can take is that I originally requested and pushed for an antipsychotic shortly after his diagnosis. Other than that, I was completely befuddled by his disorder.

When he wanted to be left completely alone in the early months after his regression, I left him alone as much as possible, until he wanted to approach us. I do not regret that, but I am not saying it was right. I have read articles promoting the provision of an almost overstimulating environment. In my opinion, this would have driven Aaron over the edge.

Every so often I ask Aaron about what he went through in the early stages of his illness, and what he is still going through. I do not question him often, because he does not like to talk about it, but I have a desperate desire to know what happened to him, so as to have some understanding of what he thought and felt. The most important thing I have learned from speaking to Aaron is that children with CDD have a visual perception problem. Remember, I am not an expert, and these views are coming from a child diagnosed with CDD. Aaron uses an example of a room suddenly looking different. The room abruptly appears to be getting smaller, with the walls coming closer to him. At other times, trees will also look different, and seem to move even when there is no wind. When we are driving, he will occasionally complain that I nearly hit a car head on, or when I pull up to the house, he will say I almost hit the tree on the lawn. For the past two summers, he refused to wear shorts. Finally this summer, he told me why. He explained that he cannot stand it when mosquitoes or flies land on his legs; he cannot feel them when he wears long pants.

At the beginning of his disorder he ate very little. Now he consumes an enormous amount of food. I cannot understand how a child his size can eat so much, but he is not overweight. I am not sure if it is a symptom of CDD, or if it is caused by his medication. He explains that he is hungry all of the time. He also explains that the compulsion he had with the face cloth—always wiping his hands and face—was because his skin constantly felt sticky and he was trying to clean it off. I wonder how many logical explanations he has for all of the odd behavior he had, or still has. I hope over time he will be able to answer all of my questions. Today, a stranger would probably not be able to ascertain that anything was wrong with Aaron. He no longer attacks people or throws food. Noise does not seem to bother him, and he enjoys a day at a noisy amusement park. Instead of going into a frenzy when the phone rings, he now answers it. He has excellent eye contact and at times talks a blue streak. In June 1996, his speech had progressed to that of a 5-year-old, with still some delay in his expressive language. In June he was 6.2 years of age, so he is catching up.

In some ways, I do not think the doctors or psychologists realize how far he has come in his speech. He will either refuse to answer their questions, or give them the quickest, shortest reply he can. On one occasion, just after we left the doctor's office, I asked him why he is so quiet while we are in the office. He told me that he hates hearing people talk about him and wants the visits short so he can go home. I explained to him that if he does not talk more in front of the doctor, the doctor will not know how well he is, and then we will have to come more often. He started talking slightly more in later visits, but not much. He still hates going to the doctor.

Aaron still has some persistent odd behaviors. He will laugh inexplicably every so often, or become extremely angry over next to nothing. He still walks on his tiptoes. He did this when he was a baby, but two of my nieces also did this. They eventually outgrew it around the kindergarten age, so I was not overly concerned. Aaron seemed to be growing out of the habit until he was struck with CDD, then the toe-walking became worse, and continues to this day. Every time I see him on his tiptoes, I remind him to walk on his feet. He does for a while, until he forgets. It is one habit I wish he could overcome. It is a physical trait that sets him apart from other, "normal" children.

If Aaron manages to learn to read and write and even has a basic concept of math, I think he can lead a generally independent life. He still has another 12 years of school, so his future does not appear too bleak. That is only if things continue as they are. My greatest fear is that

Aaron will lose the skills he has regained. His doctors admit that they have never seen another child with CDD, and are as much in the dark as I am. Throughout the past 2 years, Aaron has had several episodes of regression severe enough to be quite noticeable, but so far, these periods have not lasted more than a week or two at a time. Every time this happens, I always worry that he will not come as far back as he was before. Increasing his medication does not seem to make any difference. It is a constant cycle of two steps forward, one step back. I have no idea why this happens, but it always scares me. When I mentioned to my daughter one day that Aaron had been regressing for the past week or so, she commented that if children with CDD do not improve as much as Aaron has already, then maybe it is possible that he will lose all he has regained and stay where all of the doctors and literature say he should be. I never looked at it from that perspective before. It made me realize that we are not out of the woods yet. I think she was preparing me for the day that it could become a reality.

Several thoughts come to mind as I reflect over the past 2 years. One is how grateful I am for the support I had at the beginning of Aaron's disorder. It was a relief to talk to people about what was going on. Slowly over time, though, I think people get tired, and their support fades. I do not blame anyone for that. When something like CDD strikes your child, it is not only your child who changes; you do, also. I no longer have the time, nor the interest, in anything or anyone but Aaron. People who incessantly complain about trivial matters annoy me. Those stressed at selecting wallpaper for their kitchen have no idea what a real problem is. The one good thing that has come of Aaron's illness is that it helped me discover what is truly important in life.

I call what Aaron has an illness. I believe something attacked his brain even though medical science is not advanced enough to know what it was. A cause will probably not be discovered even during Aaron's lifetime. I am completely baffled how a child who was so healthy, who never had as much as an ear infection, could get such a rare, unexplained, horrible illness. Not knowing "why" is the hardest thing to deal with.

I remember when Aaron's psychiatrist said that CDD had many features similar to "late-onset autism." I did not know much about autism at the time, and what I did know was mostly wrong. I thought autistic kids were born that way and never had any period of normal behavior. I also thought that they were very passive, and in their own worlds all of the time. I thought the only thing they ever did was spin pot lids all day. I had no idea that they were aggressive, had other odd behavior, or had any of the multitude of symptoms Aaron displayed. There is much research occurring in the field of autism. Maybe this will lead to an answer for CDD

Over the last year, Adam and I discussed Aaron's improvements, as well as his medication, countless times. Early on, Adam was of the opinion that Aaron was improving on his own, and that the medication only helped calm him. I never believed that, and on three different occasions, we lowered his medication slowly, with the same result. Aaron regressed significantly each time. We always boosted his medication back up before he regressed too far. Today, Adam does not question the benefit of the medication. He knows it is the reason Aaron is as well as he is. Why Risperidal did not work, and why Largactil does, is a mystery. Both medications should have had the same result, but did not. It was a blessing that the first antipsychotic that Aaron was placed on had a positive effect. If he was tried on three or four different drugs with the same result as he had with Risperidal, I would have given up.

I believe another reason for Aaron's improvement was that he had only regressed for a period of 4 months before I managed to get him on Largactil. He still acquired weird behavior while on the medication, and his dose was very low to start, but I believe I caught him early enough to make a difference. He seemed to forget everything he had previously learned, but after reacquiring some speech, I began teaching him things he knew before. He gradually relearned different colors and other things. I found that what he knew previous to his illness came much quicker to him than what he did not know. Learning new material is more difficult. Before I accepted his diagnosis of CDD, I asked his doctor if he could be schizophrenic because an antipsychotic medication is helping him. "No," I was told. He explained that 4-year-olds do not get schizophrenia, and even if they did, the onset, symptoms, and course of the two disorders are different. I read what I could find on childhood schizophrenia and discovered that age 13 was considered "very early onset." Even when I found several cases of children diagnosed before the age of "very early onset," I discovered that the assessment of Aaron's doctor was consistent with medical literature. There were major differences in the two disorders, and Aaron would not fit the criteria for schizophrenia. Nonetheless, I believe that CDD, autism, and schizophrenia are all linked together in some way.

I was told by another psychiatrist that Aaron may, later in life, have his diagnosis changed to schizophrenia. Although he fit all of the criteria of CDD, because he has regained more skills than he should have, there will probably come a day when his diagnosis will be changed. I asked him what medication other CDD children were tried on. He did not know the answer. He said that because there were so few cases of CDD, it was statistically impossible to know what treatments have been tried.

We are living one day at a time with Aaron. So far, he continues to improve. He has not reached a plateau yet. There was a time when I hoped that one of his medical tests would show something abnormal, but not anymore. He had his latest EEG 3 months ago, and everything is still normal. How far he will come back has yet to be seen. For over 2 years, Aaron's life, as well as the rest of the family's, has been misery. However, things are returning to normal. I can think of other things during the day now besides Aaron. In fact, I recently wallpapered my kitchen.

I think Aaron has finally crossed over the 70 or 75% line on his return home. The way is dark, but I have the candles lit. With God's help, I hope he can make it the rest of the way.

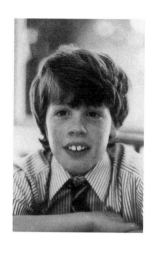

Five

Diary of David

by Jenny Fairthorne

Nedlands in suburban Perth, Western Australia, is an idyllic place to live. Not only does it bask in the same warm and sunny climate as the surrounding regions, but it is enhanced by the adjacent unspoiled and tranquil Swan River. This scenic backdrop provides a venue for riverside strolls and picnics as well as a medium for a variety of water sports. Moreover, Nedlands is central to the amenities of a city of some million people. Yet at the same time it has many of the advantages of a country town. My husband, Fred, is a successful grocery retailer. I am a secondary mathematics teacher. Our first child, Tom, was born in 1983. Two and a half years later, we were again blessed with a healthy child, a girl whom we named Sarah. Our third child is David. This is the first chapter of his story.

Monday, April 25, 1988—ANZAC Day
    ANZAC Day is a public holiday, peculiar to Australia and New Zealand. "ANZAC" is an acronym for "Australia and New Zealand Army Corps." The day is a tribute to the thousands of Australasian soldiers who died for their countries while at war. No work for Fred as his

92   WHEN AUTISM STRIKES

supermarkets were closed. It was open-house day at Penrhos College. We decided to visit.

Fred and I, along with 5-year-old Tom and 2½-year-old Sarah in a pusher, explored the plush facilities of this prestigious girls' school. Filing through a science laboratory, we came across some forgotten friends, Adam and Robyn, who had two young daughters named Megan and Jessica, who were similar in ages to Tom and Sarah. Sadly, Jessica had Down syndrome and Adam had been unable to accept this. I remember Robyn telling of the choice he had given her. Stated simply, it was, "me or the baby." So Robyn placed Jessica in foster care and visited and took her out while Adam was at work.

I could empathize with both Adam and Robyn. I wondered whether some obsession with perfection had caused Adam to initially reject his second daughter. I was grateful that fate had not placed such strains on my family.

Tuesday, June 7, 1988—Cholera/typhoid vaccination
Fred and I had decided to take a second honeymoon in Malaysia, hence the immunization appointment. On mentioning to Dr. Pearce that I might be pregnant, he pulled out an encyclopedia from his bookshelf. He read and then translated, "It's not a live vaccine. It won't cross the placenta."

Monday, June 27, 1988, 8:45 AM—Visit to Dr. Pearce
My pregnancy was confirmed with an estimated date of delivery of March 2, 1989. Fred and I were pleased as we had decided on a third child 6 months before.

Monday, February 27, 1989—In-service day at school
At 6:00 AM, it became apparent that today was to be our third child's birthday. The timing was impeccable. Tom and Sarah had no school, hence, they were available to be ferried in to meet their new sibling. My mother had arrived from Adelaide a few days earlier and was keen to mind her grandchildren. At 12:24 PM, David was born. He was a perfect child with a mass of beautiful, almost iridescent, golden hair.

Sunday, August 5, 1990, 3 PM—David Cowan's party
The five of us were in attendance at David Cowan's seventh birthday celebration. Our 17-month-old David was an enchanting, extroverted, little party animal. He loved to dance and the bigger the group and the more pronounced the beat, the more he enjoyed himself. Fred and I were very proud of our sociable toddler. Sitting on a sofa, we supervised David from afar as he moved from eating cake outside, to the dance area where he joined another dozen children. He immediately became part of the group, jumping enthusiastically to the beat of the loud music.

Monday, July 8, 1991—Fly to Tweed Heads
Fred's parents live in Tweed Heads, which is on the East Coast of Australia. The children were excited at the thought of seeing their grandparents again. Among our luggage were two violins, a cassette recorder, and a variety of Suzuki Violin Tapes. For more than 4 years, we had been a Suzuki family. At 4, Tom had begun learning Suzuki Violin and 2 years later at 3, Sarah had followed. David arrived home from hospital to the sweet strains of *Boccherini's Minuet* and as he grew it was with Suzuki Repertoire as a backdrop. Not surprisingly, David loved music and was very adept at changing tapes and playing his preferred pieces. On occasions, David would prance around the sitting room to the beat of his own rendition of *Seitz Concerto I* from the Suzuki Repertoire. Often, he would loiter nearby Tom and Sarah's practice sessions and learn the bowings by heart. A favorite chant would be "Big, big, big, big, little, little, big, big" to the tune of Suzuki's *Allegro.*
Fred's mother, Jude, took the children shopping to choose gifts. David chose a "Rigadoon Joe" doll, which quickly became known as simply "Riggie." At the time Riggie and David could comfortably swap clothes. Jude remarked that David was not to be fobbed off with a scaled-down version of Riggie, despite her best efforts in this regard.
David's preferred books were Helen Oxenbury's series entitled *Tom and Pippo.* He owned two volumes, which he took pride in "reading" out loud, page by page. David also loved puzzles and could already complete more difficult jigsaws than his nearly 6-year-old sister. A favorite was a multicolored wooden puzzle that contained, in order and

in three rows, removable letters of the alphabet. David delighted in saying the letter name, followed by a word beginning with that letter, as he correctly placed the shape into its allocated spot. "W water" enthused David as he reached for the "W" and correctly inserted it into its position. At the time he wasn't even looking at the board. "This is spooky," I remarked to Fred. My statement amazed me, why did a positive ability in my son worry me? "It's as though he learned to do this in another life," replied Fred.

Monday, December 9, 1991, 3 PM—Interview at Gumnut Montessori

David was to receive the benefits of Montessori Pre-primary Education. The interview was for the teacher, Mary-Ellen, to assess whether he was ready for the experience. "He can begin on the second day of term one," she concluded after David had shyly answered three of four questions and completed two puzzles. Later that week, as I was collecting David from Marita Road, his day-care center, an attendant, Karen, drew me aside.

"I'm concerned about David's speech," she began.

"He's got too many labels and not enough action words," she added.

I wasn't quite sure what she wanted me to do. "You're a bit hard to please," I thought. "Do you want me to start training him, and gather statistics on verb-to-noun ratios, and see if we can increase the ratio over time?" I had cynically pondered.

Tuesday, December 10, 1991—Marita Road Christmas party

David and his 2-year-old peer group at day care had been practicing their concert item for the last week. The children looked appealing in beetle costumes, and they were impatient to perform their item. Surprisingly, David was not happy to join his group and when we went to leave, he began sobbing. We decided to take him with us to watch the other items. When it was his turn to perform, we would take him to join his group. The beetles came out ready to dance; they were eagerly anticipating the carefully chosen classical music that was about to fill the air. Uncharacteristically, David was insecure and set on staying with his family. Under no circumstances was this beetle going to dance. After the concert, David's usual happy affect returned, and he was pleased to meet Father Christmas. He eagerly unwrapped his gift.

Tuesday, December 17, 1991, 8:30 AM—Audiologist
In June 1990, tiny tubes or "grommets" were inserted through David's eardrums. During the appointment, David was happy and co-operative. According to the report, he had "grommets in situ" and "Sound field responses are within normal limits."

Wednesday, December 25, 1991
The children were amazed to find a cubby house in a secluded corner of the garden. Indoors all was strangely quiet as the three children set up their new playhouse. David was a motivated participant and did not mind at all being subservient to the demands of his older brother and sister. We spotted him helping Sarah by carrying dolls' mattresses and blankets from her bedroom. Next, like Tom, he was transporting a child-sized chair.

Tuesday, December 31, 1991—Cousin Anne arrives
Within the week, 11-year-old cousin Anne had become a firm friend of David's. She and Sarah were sharing a room at the opposite end of the house from David's room. His habit was to visit the girls first thing in the morning where he would cuddle, chat, and play.
Since Karen had voiced her concerns, I had been taking particular note of David's speech. She had been right—at the time, David's speech had been telegraphic. Now, over the last month I had been gratified to observe his linguistic abilities multiply. Now, there was no shortage of verbs and along with nouns there were adjectives, adverbs, pronouns, prepositions, and so forth. All were skillfully combined in age appropriate sentences. On David's return to the day-care center, I again conferred with Karen. She confirmed that David's sentence structure and vocabulary had rapidly improved. It never occurred to me that a child's abilities could wax and wane. Apart from damage related to documented accident or disease, intellectual and emotional regression were beyond the scope of my imagination.

Saturday, January 18, 1992, 10:30 AM—Noddy at Regal Theatre
David was entranced by a performance of *Noddy* at our local the-
ater. There was a "Noddy Song" set to a catchy melody involving distinctive arm movements as the hero's name was spelled. Over the next
week, David derived immense pleasure from performing the "Noddy
Song." As he sung the letters of the hero's name, his hands and arms
would move from head to shoulders to chest, just as he had seen the
previous Saturday.

Saturday, January 25, 1992—Kays for dinner
The Kay family had joined us for a barbecue. The children were
playing when David appeared in a doorway with Sarah's violin tucked
under his arm. Purposefully, he strode until he was standing directly in
front of us and pausing, he waited for our attention. Only then did his
efforts to play begin and with violin under chin, he began to scrape at
the strings with the bow. I decided that it was time for David to begin
his Suzuki career.

Tuesday, February 4, 1992
David's preprimary education began at the Gumnut Montessori
School. There was much to learn, but he had enjoyed the day. As I
waited at the gate, I watched and listened as he shook hands and said
clearly and with a smile, "Good afternoon, Mary-Ellen." Such is the
Montessori custom. A school day ends with a handshake and appropriate parting words.

Wednesday, February 19, 1992—David's first violin lesson
David began violin lessons. Unlike my older children, David was
unfailingly keen to practice. At the appropriate time, he would
earnestly fetch his violin and accessory bag with no prompting. At this
early stage, practice consisted of learning the names of different parts of
the violin, rehearsing a correct bow hold, and bowing to an imagined
audience. The last of these tasks, David performed with his bow carefully hooked onto his right index finger and his violin tucked neatly at
waist height, under his right arm.

Sunday, March 1, 1992—David's birthday party
David had turned 3 years old on February 27, 1992. His godparents, David and Joan Coutts, were staying for the weekend to attend David's birthday party.

While I prepared breakfast, I listened for the familiar call of "Mummy" from David's room. This constituted a summons and a request for me to open his cot so that he might begin his day. I decided to wake David. He was sitting in his cot, eyes opened and yet motionless. When I entered, he appeared not to hear me, as if in a trance. Clicking my fingers only centimeters from his nose evoked no response. What strange spell had been cast on my child? Wanting a second opinion, I raced downstairs and beckoned Fred and Joan to come and observe. When the three of us arrived in the bedroom, David was sitting exactly as before, staring blankly and not responding to movement or sound. Minutes later, the prolonged trance suddenly ended. David returned to be the same extroverted, affectionate, and talkative child as before. We soon forgot about the incident. David's peculiar turns continued for the next month or so. Several mornings a week, I would enter his room and find him sitting in bed, glazed and unresponsive for maybe 2 or 3 minutes.

Thursday, April 23, 1992—Wedding rehearsal
Sarah was to be a flower girl at her cousin Tim's wedding to Lisa. David, Tom, and I waited in the pews as the bride and pastor choreographed the wedding party's entrance, wait at the altar, and exit. I was surprised that David was totally disinterested in the proceedings and asked no questions. He seemed unable to sit and watch and instead kept jumping up and trying to head for the aisle.

Sunday, April 26, 1992, 1:30 PM—Tim and Lisa's wedding
At the wedding, David kept repeating "I want to go to the toilet."

"You've just been to the toilet," I tried to reason with him. It was as though he wanted to escape from the church.

Six months later, we reviewed the videotape of the wedding and noticed that David did not reply, even though his grandmother greeted him three times. It was also surprising to note that I was grasping him very firmly by the wrist rather than simply holding his hand. "Let go. You're hurting me," David protested on tape. It was as though I was expecting him to bolt!

Monday, May 18, 1992, 5 PM—Violin party
David was elated to be included in a violin performance at his teacher's home. He walked proudly into the sitting room with his violin under his arm. While the advanced students played, David clapped enthusiastically. Three children had performed when David decided that it must now be his coveted moment. He stood up and announced, "It's my turn." With great concentration, he placed his violin and bow into exactly the right position and performed his well-practiced bow. The applause of the onlookers thrilled him.

Over the next few months, David was less placid and at times distraught for no apparent reason. He was playing his tapes more often and for longer periods. He would sit by the cassette player listening to the music as though it both comforted and entranced him.

At times, he became set on an idea and would become upset if his wishes were not granted. For example, prior to dinner one evening, David decided that he wanted us all to go to the local Greek restaurant instead of eating at home. "I want to go to Greco's," he repeatedly wailed. My explanations and consolations made little difference.

Wednesday, July 1, 1992, 12 noon—Interview with Mary-Ellen
Mary-Ellen was concerned at the deterioration of David's behavior in the classroom since term one. Increasingly, he seemed not to hear her instructions and sometimes, he would suddenly stand and run around the classroom as though confused. "He's very intelligent," she emphasized. "But I need to know if he's hearing me," she added with concern.

Friday, July 10, 1992, 8:45 AM—Child Health Centre
I was mildly worried about David but ultimately I thought that he was just having some transient problem that would resolve itself. We visited the Child Health Centre to obtain a referral to the Child Guidance Clinic, which was more specialized in dealing with the develop-

mental and emotional problems of childhood. "The appointment is only to placate Mary-Ellen," I told myself.

Wednesday, July 15, 1992—Appointment at audiologist
David's hearing was tested and reported to be well within normal range. The audiologist, Martin Wall, had explained that children who have suffered hearing loss sometimes have behavioral problems as a result of the previous deprivation. I was pleased and relieved and did not doubt this explanation for David's uncharacteristic behavior.

Saturday, July 18, 1992—Betty returns
My mother, Betty, had been overseas since Tim and Lisa's wedding in April. Vividly, I remember the moment she walked into our living room where David was perched on his father's knee. Something about David caused his grandmother to exclaim,
"He's changed!"
"Don't be ridiculous," I replied intolerantly.
"It's been 12 weeks and he's temporarily forgotten you," I added.
Now I had two reasons to push for an appointment at Child Guidance Clinic, my mother's concern as well as that of Mary-Ellen.

Monday, August 3, 1992, 3:30 PM—Assessment at Child Guidance Clinic
Fred, David, and I arrived promptly for the consultation with Sally Woods at Child Guidance Clinic. We began by relaying the concerns of Betty and Mary-Ellen.
"Does David always dribble like he is now?" asked Sally.
My immediate reaction was to answer negatively, as I thought of the David of a few months ago. But I restrained myself and thought about our changing boy.
"Not always," I answered thoughtfully. "The drooling comes for a day or so and then recedes." All at once other new behaviors came to mind. David often appeared as though he was in a trance and did not respond when I called his name.
"Last year, he had a runny noise all winter, and was on antibiotics and generally run down," reported Fred.

"David gets easily agitated and jumps up and down on the spot. Sometimes, he covers his ears with his hands as though he is hearing something which is hurting his ears," I contributed.

A major concern was discipline. In the past, I had prided myself on the good behavior and manners of my children. Now, I was at a loss because David no longer responded to the positive and negative consequences that worked so well for Tom and Sarah.

"The only way to get David to follow an instruction is to lead him through it," I told Sally. At the conclusion of the meeting, Sally said that she was going to refer us to a developmental pediatrician at the Child Development Centre in West Perth. As a social worker, she did not feel that David's problems were in her domain.

Thursday, August 27, 1992, 9 AM—Observation at Gumnut

Today, I was to sit and passively observe David at school. I was hoping to glean more insight into his expanding portfolio of bizarre behavior. As I waited, the word *autism* came to mind. "Autism is a condition where afflicted children are trapped in their own world," I recalled from a television documentary. Only once had I met an autistic child and I recalled the experience graphically. A friend and I were arriving at a fellow university student's party. The hostess, Christina, came forward to meet us. She introduced us to her brother who looked to be about 10. He smiled and looked as though he was about to speak but instead produced strange nonverbal noises. I was stunned and embarrassed. "Was this boy playing some immature prank?" Christina clearly read my confusion and hastily explained, "Aaron is autistic. Some people find his behavior rather strange." Reconciling David's behavior with Aaron's was impossible. Unlike Aaron, David could articulate and speak in perfectly constructed sentences. It was just that he had lost the desire to communicate.

It was time to go in. I walked to the back of the classroom and sat down. David had noticed and had caught my gaze. "You're not supposed to be here," he said with his eyes.

It was time for the roll call. On the carpet, the children sat in a large circle with Mary-Ellen among them.

"Rachel Ainsworth," Mary-Ellen called.

"Here," replied Rachel in a clear voice.

"Justin Arthur."

"Here," chanted Justin loudly.

"David Fairthorne."

Silence.

"David Fairthorne," repeated Mary-Ellen patiently. More silence.

"David Fairthorne," Mary-Ellen said again with the same calm-ness.

This time her assistant Merl was by David's side and with her prompting, he was able to respond correctly. A numbness emanated from within me. What had happened to my beloved son? It was as though I was dreaming. Later, I would laugh with a friend about my ir-rational nightmare. Children don't lose their minds, at least not without some obvious cause. It was an effort not to cry.

At the end of the session, I took David by the hand to fetch his hat and schoolbag. He was talking, not to me, not even to himself, but talk-ing for the sheer pleasure of the auditory sensation. I listened carefully.

"Open the fridge door. Take out the jug with two hands. Put the jug on the table and fetch a glass. . . ." David was repeating the instruc-tions he had heard when Merl was teaching him to get himself a glass of chilled water. "Why are you talking about getting a drink of water?" I asked David. But he continued his recital without responding to my question.

Thursday, September 3, 1992

By now, we were very anxious to see the developmental pediatri-cian. David's case, however, did not have any urgency associated with it and so we had to queue until it was our turn. October 5 was the date given. Meanwhile, David was losing skills and becoming increasingly difficult to manage. Trips in the car had become trials of my patience. Sitting in his seat presented grave difficulties for my now-overactive son. On one occasion, he managed to keep his seat belt fastened but his head was resting on the floor and his feet on the headrest.

"Come and see what David's doing," I called to Fred. He was sit-ting on the carpet in Sarah's room and looking through a "Tom and Pippo" book. Strangely, he was feeling the pages by sliding his hand re-peatedly up and down the page. The pictures and text that had previ-ously given him so much pleasure were locked from his perception.

"Self-stimulation," I said to Fred. "According to what I have read, autistic children self-stimulate."

In the mornings, Fred had developed the habit of taking David out with him on his bicycle. With David strapped happily into the child seat on the back, the two would ride along the bike path next to the river, singing loudly as the wind rushed past their faces. A favorite of David's for some time had been *Old MacDonald Had a Farm*. As they sped along, they would sing verses of this rhyme. David would nominate the animal and then together they would continue with the appropriate animal call. Next, Fred would be the initiator. Each day, Fred reported that David could sing a little less of the song. Each day, our fears for our son intensified.

Friday, September 25, 1992—Departure for Malaysia

Six months before, we had organized a week's holiday at Club Med in Malaysia. It was to have been the perfect family holiday. Unfortunately, our expectations and the reality were quite distinct. By now, David's grasp on reality was very impaired. Gazing with a glazed expression into perceived nothingness was an increasing preoccupation.

The resort's restaurant was elevated about 4 meters from the natural ground level. It had a roof to shade but no walls. The feeling created was of dining in a tropical garden. While in the restaurant, David was confused. The flurry of activity from the staff, the chatter of the guests, the dazzling reflections from the surrounding, moatlike swimming pool, and the movement of the adjacent foliage were all enormous distractions for him. Apart from eating, David spent much of his time in the restaurant on Fred's chair. He would crawl into the space between Fred and the backrest as though this provided him with a solace.

Saturday, October 3, 1992—Leave for home

On Monday, David was to see the developmental pediatrician. "Even if the diagnosis is horribly negative, we will be in a stronger position than we are now in our ignorance," I thought. "Having a prognosis will mean that we can plan and thereby optimize our family's lifestyle and future," my thoughts continued. "Don't expect a decision instantly," I prepared myself. "It might be a few weeks as the doctor may need to run tests," I concluded.

Monday, October 5, 1992, 11 AM—Appointment with Dr. Rowe
Fred, David, and I were to meet with Dr. Rowe, the pediatric registrar, and Judith, the senior social worker. The round-table conference began and Dr. Rowe put David through the paces of his first "Griffith's Test." Judith insisted on clapping loudly immediately behind David's back, presumably to see if he would respond. Of course, he didn't; but irritatingly, she persisted in doing it again and again.

We voiced our concerns and related how our son had changed from extroverted, articulate, and affectionate to withdrawn, silent, and confused. The collection of David's personal statistics was next on the agenda and Dr. Rowe, Fred, and David moved outside to the scales.

Within seconds of their departure, Judith began asking me questions.

"So David has three baby-sitters during a week and you are a mathematics teacher," she said.

"Each day is different for David. There's no routine," she continued.

"Who does the mothering?" the social worker finished with a flourish.

"She thinks I've abused my child," I concluded in disbelief.

When Fred, David, and the doctor returned, she became silent.

Dr. Rowe read his notes and announced, "I'm organizing a CT scan, EEG, complete blood profile, and urine metabolic screen. Blood will also be taken for chromosome testing."

"What do you think?" I asked.

"It is difficult to say, but David may have a Pervasive Developmental Disorder," Dr. Rowe replied.

"Do you think that he is autistic?" I asked.

"Let's wait for the test results and then we'll review the situation in 6 weeks," he responded.

Home we went to the challenge of continuing with our lives. The report from Dr. Rowe came and I was shocked to find that David's General Quotient from the Griffith's Test was estimated to be 79. As a former student of psychology, I recalled the common truncation point for intellectual disability of 80 points. Up until this time, I had never considered that David had lost intelligence as well as speech and social skills. But of course, he had.

Dr. Rowe telephoned with the final result. "It looks good. All of the test results are back and the nasty degenerative disorders have been eliminated."

Sunday, October 18, 1992—Picnic at King's Park

Tom, Sarah, and I organized a picnic and headed for nearby King's Park to join David's classmates and their families for lunch. I observed David closely as he played among the other children. My recent reading had added substance to my concept of autism and I was happy to find that on a number of counts David just did not fit the picture.

"Empty" said David as he stood in front of me holding a squashed box that had formerly contained "Smarties."

"You're communicating, David," I thought, "that's not characteristic of autism."

"He's very intelligent," rang Mary-Ellen's words.

"Autistic children have an average IQ of 50," echoed the words in the journal article. This statement gave me confidence because David could count and read numbers from 1 to 20, recognize the 26 letters of the alphabet, and read his favorite books by recognition. His academic achievements seemed numerous.

Despite this reassurance, the adrenaline resurfaced as I faced the perceived reality. Maybe David was not autistic but disabled socially. Had I kept him too busy? Were violin lessons, childcare, and home-help too much for a boy sensitive to change as Dr. Rowe had suggested? Had David's lifestyle precipitated his regression?

Suddenly, I felt blameworthy and underconfident. "Refrigerator mothers cause their children to withdraw from the world and become autistic." The words of the dated text from the local library taunted me.

My reflections transported me again. "Look what you've done to him," instructed Fred as he looked across the kitchen to David. As was increasingly common, David was sitting beside his cassette player and listening to yet another Suzuki tape. The music appeared to both daze and comfort him. "Why is Fred attacking me?" I thought with alarm. David bounced off the stool without warning and then ran excitedly to the CD player in the nearby living area. Within seconds, country music and Suzuki were being played simultaneously. I thought, "David doesn't love music at all. It's the noise; he can't seem to get enough auditory stimulation."

Tuesday, October 27, 1992, 8:15 AM—Meeting at Christ Church School
We had intended to send David to Nedlands Primary School with his brother and sister. As the hint of a disability began to balloon, I realized that the best place for David might be Christ Church Grammar School. This school was well known for the way it supported boys with mild disabilities and in addition it had an Education Support Centre for boys with tested intellectual disability. "Of course, David won't need that level of support," I reassured myself.

Today, Fred and I met Harold Woodall, the school registrar. Proudly, Harold showed off the chapel, the swimming pool, the music and drama suites and the light, airy classrooms.

"Please can we see the Support Unit?" I asked hesitantly.

"Is your son disabled?" asked a puzzled Harold.

"We're not sure," answered Fred.

"He might need some extra help," I tacked on.

We left with forms to complete. A place in Year One in 1995 could be secured with the payment of a term's fees.

"David's admission to the Education Support Unit would require special consideration by the headmaster and the head of the Special Education Department," Harold told us. I decided to acquire the Year One place for David and then, if necessary, pursue the place in the Support Unit at a later date.

Monday, November 2, 1992—Conference with Geoff Matthews
Today we met Geoff Matthews, headmaster of the Preparatory School of Christ Church Grammar School. Geoff was direct and broadminded and did not falter when I mentioned that David might have some disability. The interview finished with the agreement to contact the school in the middle of 1994. We would then bring David to an interview and his needs would be assessed.

Tuesday, November 3, 1992, 9 AM—Rosalind Thomson
Speech therapist Rosalind Thomson had been recommended by Dr. Rowe to assist David's speech redevelopment. The therapy room was a paradise for David. Books lined the walls and he quickly tracked down a copy of his beloved *Very Hungry Caterpillar.*

Carefully, he opened the book to the first page.

"Moon," he commented.

He turned a few more pages and said "caterpillar."

I questioned my memory.

"Did David really tell the story page by page at the beginning of the year?"

"Please, God, tell me what has happened to my son?" I silently pleaded.

After the session, we visited Betty. As we turned into Mooro Drive, I almost expected David to cry out excitedly, "Nanna, Nanna."

"He no longer loves his grandmother," I surmised sadly.

On arrival, David would always rush to the kitchen to fetch Betty's lolly jar. Now, he burst in and instead headed for the portable radio that was within full view of the hallway. I was puzzled. David certainly still loved sweets. A new hypothesis dawned. "Was memory impairment a symptom of this syndrome that David had acquired?" I led him to the study where Betty's collection of framed family photographs was displayed. Pointing at a wedding portrait of Tim and Lisa, I asked, "Who's this, David?" He looked but seemed unable to answer my question. I asked again.

"Tim and Lisa," he replied very slowly and almost inaudibly.

"It's as though it hurts David to talk," I commented to my mother.

Thursday, November 26, 1992, 1:30 PM—Psychologist
Judith Thompson was a psychologist at the Child Development Centre where we had seen Dr. Rowe a few weeks before. He and his supervisor, Dr. Parry, had organized a consultation with her. "David sat on his mother like an armchair" and "David presented to me as a retarded, passive, autistic child," wrote Judith in her report.

All correct observations, I was sure. "Why doesn't she place any significance on David's promising earlier development? Only 5 months ago, Mary-Ellen was stressing his intelligence," I puzzled. "If a brain stopped functioning normally, then something must have changed within the brain. Efforts to find a cause for the loss of functioning might prove fruitful and treatable," I reasoned.

My reading around the subject of autism had continued, and many times I was relieved to read that one criterion for autism was "onset before 30 months."

"You don't have that, David," I would think to myself.

Monday, November 30, 1992, 10 AM—Drs. Parry and Rowe

We were to meet with Dr. Rowe again, along with the well-known Dr. Parry for the first time. I remembered Dr. Parry from posters I had read at the local Child Health Centre. Annually, he gave lectures to new parents on the trials and joys of child-rearing. I felt confident that this doctor would correctly diagnose my son. "Hello, David, and good morning, Mr. and Mrs. Fairthorne," greeted Dr. Parry. "We have decided to sit and observe David without intervention," he added.

I glanced across his desk to the large jar of jellybeans and then to the cassette player. "You're going to enjoy this, David," I thought. So Fred and I, along with Drs. Parry and Rowe, sat back and watched in silence. David moved quickly from puzzles to books to the tap on the sink. Next was the desk and David began dialing a number on the telephone. Without thinking, I intervened and took David back to the puzzles.

"We decided to observe David without intervention," said Dr. Parry. I immediately returned to my seat, embarassed that I had not managed to follow such a simple instruction. The consultation continued and the doctors looked at David and chatted to each other. "I don't think that he has Pervasive Developmental Disorder," said Dr. Parry to Dr. Rowe.

That sounded positive. From my reading, I had gleaned that children who did not present positively on enough criteria to be diagnosed as autistic would often be left with the less severe label of PDD. So just as a quadrilateral cannot be a square if it's not a rectangle, I concluded that if David did not meet the criteria for PDD, then he could not possibly meet the criteria for autism.

"I think that he's autistic," finished Dr. Parry.

I gasped.

Dr. Parry turned to us and said, "You may wish to contact Mildred Creak Centre, which is the support service financed by the State Government for autistic children."

Without waiting for a reply, he added, "I will make the necessary arrangements."

As Fred and I walked toward the car with David, it felt as though my life had hit its lowest ebb.

"I can't handle this, Fred, it's too much," I sobbed.

"You're just going to have to," responded Fred.

Within a few days, Dr. Parry's report arrived. "The mild degree of his differences, though they are clearly present, suggest the possibility of Asperger's syndrome. There is no evidence of true deterioration" was the conclusion. I was stunned. Dr. Parry simply did not believe that David had been a bright, extroverted, and healthy child.

Wednesday, December 2, 1992, 3 PM—Jura Tender

Jura Tender was a psychologist at the Mildred Creak Centre. She was to provide us with information and counseling.

"A Lovaas Intervention Programme would help David. Forty-nine percent of autistic children who undergo Lovaas Intervention recover from autism," she informed us with conviction.

I looked at Fred. There was no doubt in our minds, we would organize such a program for David. A 49% chance of retrieving our child sounded unbelievably good.

"How do we start?" I asked. Jura thought for a few moments of the names of therapists.

"Phone Jenny Bolland," was her instruction.

Wednesday, December 9, 1992, 10:30 AM—Jenny Bolland

It had been reassuring to speak with Jenny a few days earlier. She had not only sounded sympathetic but very knowledgeable and experienced in the area of Lovaas Intervention with preschool autistic children. For the last 2 years, she had been employed by Murdoch University to supervise the Young Autism Project. This was to be a replication of the work of Ivar Lovaas at the University of California in Los Angeles. Jenny was keen to "work with David," as she put it. With an intervention program, Jenny was confident that David could be taught many skills. I loved her quiet respect for him.

We arranged for Jenny to tailor a program for David. For 6 days a week, there would be 2½ hour morning and afternoon sessions. Along with Jenny, trained volunteers, Tina and Corinna, would conduct sessions. Meanwhile, I was to advertise in the local paper for more people to be trained to work with David in this intensive intervention program. I felt a surge of relief. If we tried hard enough, we might conquer this insidious and mysterious disorder yet.

Thursday, December 10, 1992, 9 AM—Intervention session
Today David was to start his intervention program. Jenny was to conduct the session and Fred and I were to observe. Tomorrow evening we were to undergo training in the Lovaas technique. The program seemed well organized and sensible. Jenny had divided up David's working time into a number of categories. Each of these categories was comprised of tasks. The categories were: Object Identification, Verbal Instructions, Directed Play, Undirected Play, Fine Motor Skills, and Gross Motor Skills.

To Tom and Sarah's disappointment, their playroom was to become a classroom for David. Initially, a majority of the learning tasks were to utilize a child-sized table and chairs and various equipment kept in the room. For example, Riggie, David's large doll, was the leading prop in a verbal instruction task. "Kiss Riggie," Jenny would command. Sometimes David would respond correctly and Riggie would receive a kiss on his cheek.

Fred and I watched with intrigue as Jenny led David through his first session. One task in the category of Object Identification required David to choose an item. On the tabletop, she placed a toy car and a shoe.

"Give me the shoe," drilled Jenny.

David picked up the car and handed it to Jenny.

"I don't get it!" I exclaimed.

"David knows these words, why we've even got him on video referring to his sandals." With a rush, I came to understand another facet of David's regression. Not only had David lost speech but to a large degree, he had lost the ability to understand speech.

"Acquired verbal auditory agnosia with severe reduction in spontaneous oral expression" was how I was later to hear these symptoms described.

Saturday, January 2, 1993
We planned a trip to Melbourne 10 months ago for all five of us to attend the Suzuki Pan-Pacific Conference. Now, David's violin lessons had ceased as he no longer possessed the level of cognitive functioning required. Sadly, Tom, Sarah, and I bade farewell to Fred and David. David was now committed to more than 35 hours of intervention per week.

Wednesday, January 13, 1993
Today was Day One in terms of my revised interaction with David and I was keen to apply my newly acquired Lovaas techniques to teaching David and managing his behavior in a more effective and relaxed manner. A pleasant stroll from our home is a children's playground. With David on my left and a magazine in my right hand, I set off for this planned destination with high hopes. On arrival, David headed for the climbing net and I decided to sit on a log bordering the sandpit and peruse David and the magazine concurrently. It worked well for 30 seconds! By this time, David had targeted the nearby river. He was halfway there when I noticed that he had abandoned the climbing frame.

Dropping the magazine, I darted after him but he was so fast that he was paddling in ankle-deep water by the time that I reached him.

"No harm in ankle-deep water," I told myself, trying determinedly to stay composed and relaxed. David paddled for a minute or two and then I realized that the water was now gently lapping above his knees.

"I'll take off his shorts and T-shirt so that he can have a good paddle in the knee-deep water," I thought.

I looked across at a pair of seagulls who had just landed on the nearby jetty. I glanced back at David. He was immersed to his neck and bobbing up and down, desperately trying to tread water.

"My new strategy is totally unviable," I thought as I strode through the water to rescue David.

Monday, April 5, 1993, 4 PM—Dr. Walsh

Today we were to meet with Dr. Walsh, one of Perth's three pediatric neurologists. It had suddenly come to me one afternoon that despite the fact that my son had a severe brain disorder, I had yet to consult a specialist in this area. In addition, I had read that autistic children sometimes exhibited abnormal levels of the neurotransmitter dopamine. I was keen to see if this area might be explored and treated. In short, I was slowly emerging from the shock of David's regression and my rationale was urging me to pursue possible etiologies for my son's regression.

David had been undergoing intensive Lovaas-style intervention for more than 4 months now. Initially, there had been some small gains in language but now it seemed that he had begun to regress again. New self-stimulatory behaviors were continuing to surface. Hand-flapping and licking of inedibles were now in the repertory.

David sat on the floor next to a bookcase and proceeded to remove the contents. "What can I do for you?" said Dr. Walsh.

I delivered a condensed version of David's regression.

"Would you please arrange for David to have his dopamine level tested?" I asked.

"I read in this article that autistic children sometimes have disturbed levels of dopamine."

Tuesday, April 6, 1993

It was lunchtime at Seton College and I was sitting in the Staff Room and chatting as I was eating.

"Did you watch *A Current Affair* last night?" said Simon, head of the English Department.

I shook my head and he continued.

"Lesley said that a child was featured who reminded her of David." I felt a surge of excitement.

"I was in the next room but she said that this boy lost speech at 3 and was diagnosed as autistic. It turned out that he had a rare type of epilepsy which apparently can be cured by some sort of operation."

"Do you remember what the disorder is called?" I asked with intensity. He did not.

The siren went and I returned to class. With difficulty, I contained the thrill of this new lead and directed my mind back to the graphing of parabolas.

"I'll ask Fred to get the footage," I thought.

"He advertises with Channel 9 so he'll have a useful contact."

The next evening Fred arrived home with a videocassette under his arm.

"Don't get your hopes up. This child will probably be nothing like David," I cautioned myself. "After all, Lesley has never met David and descriptions can be misleading."

The music of a recent Billy Joel song played softly in the background as the presenter told of 5-year-old Joel Huddlestone.

"After 3 years of normal development, the mother reported that Joel hallucinated and then changed dramatically. He lost both receptive and expressive language skills, interest in other people, and play skills. His favorite pastimes were now running about the backyard of his home with a watering can, and trampolining."

"This boy has the same disorder as David," I said to Fred.

"Even the age of onset is the same," he replied.

We listened on.

"Against all odds, Eva Huddlestone has discovered the disorder which afflicts her son."

This was enthusing.

"Joel has a rare form of epilepsy called Landau–Kleffner syndrome and an operation in Chicago will give him a chance to live a normal life."

This was even more enthusing and I decided to ring Eva in the morning. I awoke early and made a list of questions for Eva.

"How is LKS diagnosed?"

"Was Joel ever diagnosed as autistic?"

"Is this disease inherited?"

I was delighted when Eva answered the phone. Not surprisingly, she said that about 10 families from around Australia had contacted her.

"Landau–Kleffner syndrome is diagnosed by EEG," was her first answer.

"David's EEG was normal," I said with disappointment.

"Don't let that put you off. A normal EEG on one day might reveal seizure the next. Also, the epileptic activity may be so deep within the brain that it doesn't register on the EEG at all. I would request an extended, sleep-deprived EEG with amitriptyline as the sedative. Sometimes, commonly used sedatives such as chloral hydrate actually mask the abnormal activity." She continued, "Getting Joel diagnosed was tough. I had to send the EEG tracing to Dr. Morrell in Chicago for a positive diagnosis. The doctors here kept insisting that Joel was autistic."

It was a relief to hear that the disorder was not considered genetic. I certainly didn't want to think that it might recur in the family again. We ended our conversation with Eva offering to send a packet of information pertaining to LKS and giving me the telephone numbers of Jane Rudick and Richard Lawler. Jane was from Alabama and the mother of a child who recovered from LKS following surgery at the age of 7 years. Richard Lawler was a friend of the Huddlestones and he was in the process of forming a Support Network for the Australian parents of children with LKS or associated disorders.

Thursday, April 8, 1993

I wanted to arrange for David to undergo an extended, sleep-deprived EEG with amitriptyline as soon as possible. Not only did a diagnosis of LKS sound more likely for David on account of his prolonged early, normal development, but such a diagnosis seemed to be more positive in terms of prognosis for David. The *A Current Affair* segment had also included a clip of the recovered 9-year-old Cameron Rudick. Promisingly, his regression at age 3 had closely paralleled David's. Perth has a geographically isolated population of a little more than 1 million. Since the first documentation of LKS in 1957, there have been fewer than 100 reported cases. Considering these two factors, I was surprised to hear from Dr. Walsh that he had treated two children with the disorder. "From my experience, children with Landau–Kleffner don't present as autistic. They want to communicate and rely heavily on gesture," he said.

"We have a videotape of a child with Landau–Kleffner syndrome. He behaves in a very similar manner to David and he was originally diagnosed as autistic," I replied.

"I would be very interested to see it," said Dr. Walsh.

Hopefully, we would also be able to show him the tape of David before his regression. Then he might realize that we were realists and not parents who were not coming to terms with their son's autism.

Saturday, April 10, 1993, 9 AM—Dr. Walsh
I passed Dr. Walsh some copies of information on LKS that Eva had sent me. References pertinent to my request had carefully been highlighted.

"Prolonged EEG tracings may be necessary to uncover abnormalities."

"Many of these children may exhibit normal EEG's and the disorder is only discovered during an extended sleep-deprived recording."

"It is usually the autistic behaviours that parents find most difficult to deal with." "Amitriptyline is not commonly used for EEG testing but has recently been found to enhance abnormal activity in contrast to other sedatives which may actually mask it."

To our delight, Dr. Walsh consented to request for the extended EEG with amitriptyline as a sedative.

Monday, April 12, 1993—Taffy Reed
Several days before, Richard Lawler had told me of Taffy Reed. She was a student at Murdoch University who was studying the differences between LKS and autistic children as a thesis for her master's degree.

"There's another disorder with symptoms similar to LKS. It's called 'Childhood Disintegrative Disorder,' " she said.

Tuesday, April 13, 1993
The Lovaas program was treating David's behaviors and attempting to teach him new skills, but were we just addressing the symptoms of an underlying neurological disease? Maybe this was the best we could do but I wanted to try to find an etiology for David's autistic condition. Hopefully, this would lead to successful treatment and even cure.

A search at the medical library of the local university led me to Dr. Volkmar of Yale University. He had published an article in 1992 entitled "Childhood Disintegrative Disorder: Issues for DSM-IV." His aim was to have the disorder listed in the fourth volume of the *Diagnostic and Statistical Manual,* which provides a comprehensive list of disorders and their criteria for diagnosticians. The current volume, I later discovered, was scheduled to be superseded in May 1994. My pulse quickened as I scanned the article. For the first time I felt as though I was reading about David:

> CDD is characterized by the presence of a clearly normal period (at least 2 years) of development prior to the onset of the disorder which is associated with the loss of previously acquired skills in several areas of development and by the development of abnormal social, communicative, and behavioral functioning. The onset of the disorder may be insidious or abrupt. Premonitory signs can include increased activity levels, irritability, and anxiety, which are followed by a loss of speech and other skills. Usually the loss of skills reaches a plateau and some limited improvement may occur. In other instances the loss of skills is progressive; this is more likely when the disorder is associated with a progressive neurological condition. CDD was compared to late-onset autism. All of the children who met the proposed criteria for the disintegrative disorder had progressed developmentally to the point of using sentences prior to their developmental regression.

Of the late-onset autistic group, he reported, "None of these children had progressed developmentally past the point of using single words or phrases." Later, he compared late-onset autistic, classically autistic, and disintegrative disorder children. "The groups differed in IQ, with the disintegrative disorder group exhibiting the lowest IQ and the later onset group the higher mean IQ." I felt as though poor David had won the wrong lottery when I read of the estimated incidence of 1 in 100,000 among males.

My decision to search for an etiology was reinforced when I read that the condition had been observed in association with a number of diseases of the brain. Clinical distinctions were drawn between progressive and static forms of the disorder.

"What if David hasn't finished regressing?" I had said to Fred dismally a few months ago. To some extent my fears were proving to be grounded. David's speech had continued to decline and new autistic-like behaviors were still being manifest. Spinning plates was now a popular pastime of David's. In addition, toileting skills were becoming confused with David urinating and defecating in inappropriate venues. Nowadays it was not uncommon for David to climb out of bed in the morning and to immediately relieve himself on the carpet.

Friday, April 23, 1993, 4 PM—EEG at Princess Margaret Hospital
To my disappointment, I discovered that Dr. Walsh had changed his mind about using amitriptyline and David was not sedated during the EEG. Extended testing did not eventuate either as the recording lasted only about 2 hours. The results of David's EEG described a slight abnormality in the left temporal lobe. This was comprised of occasional spike waves and an intermittent asymmetry from the temporal region.

Dr. Walsh suggested that David undergo magnetic resonance imaging (MRI) of the brain to rule out the possibility of a tumor. I requested that David be given a second EEG this time with amitriptyline and for an extended period. Dr. Walsh agreed to organize both tests.

Friday, May 7, 1993, 3 PM—EEG at PMH
Dr. Walsh had supplied me with a prescription and I was to administer the amitriptyline an hour before David was scheduled in the hospital for the EEG. My hopes of a diagnosis were dashed when I collected David that evening. The technician reported that the results were identical to before and not supportive of a diagnosis of LKS.

"Often it is only persistent parents and doctors who arrive at a diagnosis of LKS." Eva's words interrupted my thoughts and gave me the encouragement to continue.

Thursday, May 13, 1993
I decided to write a dossier that would comprise an ordered and detailed account of David's developmental history and medical testing. Concurrently, I would organize consultations with recommended pediatric neurologists in the more densely populated east coast of Australia. If necessary, I would continue my search by consulting with recommended people on an international level. I would also send copies of the dossier to people such as Dr. Volkmar. Maybe we would get a provisional diagnosis by mail.

As an adjunct to the dossier, I decided to edit and combine onto one tape all of the footage of David before his regression. Recent footage of David after his regression would then be added to complete the picture.

Thursday, June 10, 1993, 5:30 PM—Dr. Walsh
We met with Dr. Walsh to discuss David's MRI. He began by reading the report to us. "There is a less than 1 cm linear focus of increased signal intensity in the periventricular white matter of the left frontal lobe. This may represent either a small venous angioma or a very small island of heterotopic grey matter. . . . The described white matter focus is of doubtful clinical relevance," continued the report.

Dr. Walsh explained, "This sounds like a migration abnormality. This type of defect occurs during the second trimester of pregnancy and autopsy has found heterotopia in a number of autistic children. It would seem likely that heterotopia is present throughout David's brain but the MRI has only managed to detect the largest example," he continued. "Why not come back in 5 years' time, by then our imaging techniques will have improved."

Waiting 5 years did not seem plausible to us. I was confused. On the one hand, the report placed only doubtful clinical relevance to the focus whereas Dr. Walsh suggested that it could be indicative of similar but smaller foci throughout David's brain. If a migration defect was causing David's autism, why did it not cause any apparent problem before he turned 3?

Monday, June 21, 1993—Deadline for David's history
By now, I had arranged consultations with specialists on the East Coast. Melbourne was our first stop where we had appointments with Drs. Ian Hopkins and Lloyd Shield. Then we would continue on to Sydney where we were to meet Drs. Peter Procopis and Grahame Wise. I posted a copy of the 30-page dossier and video to each of these pediatric neurologists in the hope that they would become closely acquainted with David's case before they met him in 3 weeks.

Tuesday, June 29, 1993, 11 AM—Dr. Parry
This appointment had been arranged to repeat the initial Griffith's Test that Dr. Rowe had administered the previous October. In addition, I intended to ask Dr. Parry if he considered CDD to be a plausible diagnosis for David. "The disorder is not listed in DSM IIIR so I am unable to comment," said Dr. Parry.

"He would pick up objects and constantly mouth them as though to taste before performing the task," wrote Dr. Parry of David.

No doubt this new behavior had caused him to abandon his previous suggestion that David exhibited Asperger's syndrome.

I compared the two sets of scores. Apart from the Hearing and Speech subscore, performance levels were either maintained or improved. With respect to Hearing and Speech, David's October score of 31.5 months had dropped to 22 months. It was some consolation that we were soon to receive the opinion of four other specialists.

Over the ensuing weeks, I sent copies of David's dossier and video to more than a dozen experts throughout the world. These were the pediatric neurologists who had written the journal articles telling of children who had similar presentations and histories to David. My first inquiry went to Dr. Thierry Deonna, a Swiss doctor who had written an article entitled "Acquired Epileptic Frontal Syndrome." He described a small group of children and said, "Many of the symptoms seen in our children resemble those in the developmental disorders known as 'Disintegrative Psychosis.' " He concluded his reference to CDD with "Frontal Lobe Syndrome could be one of the causes of this pattern of regression."

Next on the list was Dr. Fred Volkmar and then Dr. Lewis Rosenbloom from Liverpool. In 1978, an article coauthored by Dr. Rosenbloom had been published under the title of "Disintegrative Psychosis in Children." Ten children were described, all of whom had a similar history and clinical presentation to David. As did Dr. Volkmar, he mentioned occasional association with recognizable degenerative disorders of the nervous system.

I calculated that the children in Dr. Rosenbloom's study must now be past 20 years of age. In my letter, I asked, "Have you published any further articles which follow the development of these children?" The outcome of the development of these particular children might provide us with a prognosis for David's future.

Monday, July 12, 1993, 11 AM—Dr. Shield

After examination of David, Dr. Shield reported, "The physical examination is unremarkable apart from macrocephaly. David's head circumference is 55 cm—over the 98th percentile." I had noted this in David's dossier where I had graphed this statistic at six monthly intervals since birth. Up to the age of 12 months, David's circumference was between the 50th and 90th percentile. From 1 to 3 years, it had risen and was in the range between the 90th and 97th percentile. Shortly after age 3, the estimated age of onset of the disorder, the graph climbed more steeply. At 4½, it was well above the 98th percentile.

In closing, he suggested that David undergo a skin biopsy and urine testing for mucopolysaccharidosis and DNA testing for fragile X syndrome. These tests would eliminate additional progressive neurological disorders of childhood.

Tuesday, July 13, 1993, 9:15 AM—Dr. Hopkins

During his examination, Dr. Hopkins reported, "My feeling is that David has autistic traits which are seen in a variety of brain degenerative disorders including the Landau–Kleffner syndrome. If in spite of further evaluations a diagnosis is not reached, I think that it would be very reasonable to give diagnostic trials of both gamma globulin and corticosteroids." For the first time, a nonbehavioral treatment was suggested! It felt like a leap forward.

Thursday, July 15, 1993—Meetings with Drs. Procopis and Wise

Of David, Dr. Procopis wrote, "If not the Landau-Kleffner Syndrome, then it is likely that he has some other progressive condition affecting the speech centres predominantly. I do not believe that he has the psychiatric syndrome of autism."

"My overall impression is of a person with a progressive neurological illness," said Dr. Wise after he had carefully considered David's case.

Toward the end of each of the consultations of the last week, I had asked a question along the lines of, "Whom should we consult if we wish to pursue a diagnosis on an international level?" Considering that three of the doctors gave two names in response, I was surprised to end with only three names on my list. These were Drs. Aicardi, De Vivo, and Rapin.

I was gratified with our trip. All four doctors had raised the possibility of additional investigations and three did not believe David to be autistic. Pleasingly, one had given two suggestions for treatment.

Moreover, the foundations of our overseas quest were laid. Now I had the task of contacting Dr. Jean Aicardi in France and Drs. Darryl De Vivo and Isabelle Rapin in New York.

Monday, July 19, 1993, 8 AM—Dr. Constantinou

Dr. Constantinou was another of Perth's pediatric neurologists. He listened closely as we related the story of David's decline yet again. In pursuing a hypothesis of epileptic regression, he suggested a SPECT scan. From my understanding, this testing technique might reveal any abnormalities of blood flow within the brain. These abnormalities are often associated with seizure foci. His second suggestion was that David undergo overnight video EEG monitoring. At the conclusion of the consultation, I asked him to recommend an overseas specialist. Without hesitation, he replied, "Dr. Aicardi, he's the best." Then he added, "Dr. Cesare Lombroso and Dr. Gregory Holmes were my professors at Harvard. You might want to contact them as well. They are both epileptologists like me."

Tuesday, July 20, 1993, 12 noon—Lions' Hearing Centre

Coincidentally, David's appointment at Lions' Hearing Centre was almost exactly a year after our first consultation there with Martin Wall. His report provided an objective assessment of David's regression over the last year. Mr. Wall wrote of his observations, "His abilities have deteriorated significantly and tragically between the two occasions. He was unable to perform any of the tasks previously possible and showed no evidence of other than signal level hearing."

Wednesday, July 28, 1993

I was surprised to receive a letter from Dr. Deonna as I had only posted my package to him 3 weeks before. The letter read, "Disintegrative Psychosis is the name usually given to the disorder which David presents. It is probably not one single disease and it is possible that a very special kind of epileptic regression is the cause in some cases, and in my opinion this could be the case with David." Antiepileptic drugs were his first suggestion for treatment. It felt reassuring to hear hopeful words from another expert in the narrow field of David's rare disorder.

Saturday, August 7, 1993, 9:30 AM—Meeting with Kwong
   I decided to bring David to a friend named Kwong, who is an ear, nose, and throat surgeon, as I wanted him to organize brainstem evoked response (BSER) testing. Apparently, this is the most accurate way to assess hearing in autistic-like children. During the consultation, Kwong told us of a child whom he had examined recently. The parents, thinking that their son had been struck by sudden deafness, had initially even had him fitted with hearing aids. BSER testing later showed that his hearing was normal. After a brief pursuit of LKS, the child was given a diagnosis of autism.

Friday, August 13, 1993
   I brought David to Dr. Lam, a pediatric ophthalmologist, for a consultation in response to suggestions by Drs. Wise and Procopis, both of whom had suggested that David undergo a dilated fundus examination. A normal result would exclude further neurological diseases of childhood. David's writhing and kicks quickly halted Dr. Lam's attempts to examine his eyes. "He will need a general anesthetic for this procedure," concluded the doctor. Next on my list was to organize the skin biopsy that had been suggested by the same two neurologists. As with the ophthalmological procedure, this would exclude additional degenerative disorders of the brain.

Monday, August 23, 1993
   Today, I learned that David's DNA testing for fragile X syndrome and his urine analysis for mucopolysaccharidosis had both yielded normal results. I felt relief, particularly on the second count as mucopolysaccharidosis is an untreatable progressive disorder that almost always results in death before age 20.

Tuesday, August 24, 1993
   Dr. Constantinou concluded that the overnight video EEG recording was normal as there was only one bitemporal sharp wave during the entire recording and behavioral events such as clenching and staring had no seizure correlates.

Tuesday, August 31, 1993

Today David was to have both the skin biopsy and ophthalmological examination at Princess Margaret Hospital in Perth. Dr. Lam later reported that both results were normal. "I am sorry that David's going to have a scar on his outer wrist but Dr. Walsh particularly wanted hair follicles included. I placed the incision so that the scar will be covered by a watch," he added.

It was difficult to imagine David regaining a concept of time, but imagining him able to read a watch now felt beyond the scope of my wildest dreams. However, I simply replied to Dr. Lam, "It would be wonderful if David could one day use a watch."

Friday, September 3, 1993

My present project was planning the itinerary for our overseas trip. I began by writing to Dr. Aicardi.

Saturday, September 4, 1993

CANDLE, acronym for "childhood aphasia, neurological disorders, Landau–Kleffner, and epilepsy," is also the name of the support group directed by Jane Rudick. Some months ago, I had written to Jane and she had responded with a letter telling me of Esther Cohen in New York. Jane reported that Esther's son, Benjamin, had recently had surgery for LKS and his EEG had exhibited "not much abnormal activity in the temporal lobe." This description was reminiscent of David's recordings.

Esther was delighted to tell me the details of Ben's history and of her pathway to a diagnosis and treatment for him. Dr. Devinsky of New York University Medical Center had been her first step. While under the care of this doctor, Ben had 5 days of video EEG recording.

Monday, September 6, 1993

What an exciting day! I received a fax from London from Dr. Jean Aicardi. There was good news when I read the fax. He was to attend an Epilepsy Congress in Melbourne in November.

"I will have time to see you on November 10th," he wrote.

I was ecstatic and immediately faxed back a confirmation of the appointment.

Tuesday, September 7, 1993
Over the last year, it had become increasingly difficult to enjoy our weekends. Saturdays and Sundays had become the hardest days of the week. Not only was David's sleep cycle increasingly short but his toileting skills had become unreliable. During the week, it was easier to cope as at half past eight we could escape to the comparative relaxation of our employment. Many times, I remembered arriving at school feeling as though I had attended an all night party the night before. A party minus the fun and relaxation, that is.

The previous Sunday morning, Fred and I had been awakened at around three o'clock by an excited and giggly David. He was almost bursting with energy and trampolining fiercely on his bed. Feces and urine soiled the carpet and sheets and downstairs the kitchen had been raided. An empty bottle of lemonade was abandoned in the center of the floor and a half-empty container of melted ice cream stood next to it. We tossed for jobs. I felt lucky to score the bedroom cleanup as I knew that I was much too sleepy and grumpy to handle David. This boy was ready and determined to begin his day. Fred had the task of washing him and then trying to induce sleep. The day provided little relaxation for us or quality time with our other children. Not only were we unrested but it was essential that we were constantly vigilant. David was quick and keen to escape. Running on the road, eating soap, leaves, or dirt, climbing onto the top of first floor level balustrades—one could only guess as to what feat David might next aspire.

Family outings were now a strain on us all. One of us was always appointed as active supervisor of David but a moment's distraction was enough time for David to grab ice cream from an unsuspecting toddler's hand or to break loose from a tight grip on his wrist. I realized that I must change the format of our week. We needed to maintain the quality of our individual lives, our marriage, and our family life. Hence, I telephoned a number of support agencies. Regular weekend respite would provide us with the break from David that we urgently needed.

My first appointment was with Sherrie, the supervising social trainer of the Respite Unit at Mildred Creak Centre. She told me that weekend respite would be available every 4 or 5 weeks. The house was impressive. It was clean, spacious, and very much like a large family home. Each of the eight accommodated children slept in a bedroom with one other child. Meals were cooked and served in a large kitchen and indoor recreation was provided in a large sitting room that was furnished with armchairs, sofa, television, and boxes of toys. Outside was a large fenced and turfed area complete with a large trampoline and playground equipment. The ratio of children to staff was two to one during the day and was increased to four to one during the night. A small bus was used to take the children on a variety of outings. "Lunch at McDonald's, a picnic in the park, a trip to an adventure playground are some of the things we have done with the children," related Sherrie. I was impressed and requested that the list of families using respite be extended to include our name.

Thursday, September 9, 1993
Today, I received my second overseas fax. Dr. Isabelle Rapin had reviewed the dossier containing David's history, viewed the video, and written a two-and-a-half page report:

1. I do not believe that he has a progressive degenerative disease of the brain.
2. His case falls under the rubric of disintegrative psychosis, a poorly understood group of conditions, most of which are associated with paroxysmal EEGs with or without clinical seizures.

Treatments she suggested were steroids and anticonvulsants. "He has autistic symptoms that need treatment," she wrote.

I was encouraged and noted how closely her opinion concurred with that of Dr. Deonna. Her last sentence expressed a special interest in children such as David: "Any help you can give me by providing information on David is of vital interest to me."

Unfortunately, we were not to meet Dr. Rapin. "I see absolutely no reason for you to go to the expense and disruption of coming to the States because I could add little beyond what I can gather from the material you submitted," she explained.

Friday, September 10, 1993, 1 PM—Dr. Walsh
I brought copies of the reports that Drs. Deonna and Rapin had sent to this appointment with Dr. Walsh. Their common hypothesis of epileptic regression and suggestion of treatment using an anticonvulsant had brought me back to Dr. Walsh for his opinion and hopefully a prescription so that treatment could start immediately.

Vigabatrin was the medication specified by Dr. Walsh and David had his first dose that evening.

Wednesday, September 22, 1993
Gerard McCann was an architect who had designed our garden and today we offered him a new project. Our idea was to build a flat on top of the garage. We would then employ a person to live in the flat and help care for David. The biggest problem in our management of David was still achieving adequate sleep. If necessary, we planned to use the flat as a respite facility with David sleeping over with a caretaker.

Tuesday, October 5, 1993
David underwent a SPECT scan today. Disappointingly, the results were normal and provided no further direction for treatment or clues as to etiology.

Wednesday, October 27, 1993
The previous day, I had faxed Dr. Devinsky a request for an appointment for David during the first week of December. Today, an appointment was confirmed and in addition he suggested, "Since you are coming from so far, I believe it would be useful for you to also see Dr. Edwin Kolodny who is an international expert on developmental disorders, especially those with a genetic or metabolic basis, as well as Dr. Ruth Nass, who is a pediatric neurologist with a special interest in language development." He also wrote, "I believe that a brief video-EEG monitoring study (lasting 2–3 days) would be worthwhile." We now had two more experts to see and the opportunity to organize the extended EEG study that I had been unsuccessful in securing locally.

Thursday, October 28, 1993

My request for a quote on costs was answered. The estimate for 5 days of video monitoring was a doctor's fee of $11,575 and a hospital fee of $10,000 combining to make a particularly grand total of U.S. $21,575. I was astonished; a teacher in Australia on the top salary scale would need 9 months to earn this amount (before tax)!

We decided to book the monitoring. The itinerary of appointments for our trip to the United States had taken shape.

Monday	Dec. 6	Dr. Kolodny, NYU Medical Center
Tuesday	Dec. 7	Dr. De Vivo, Columbia Presbyterian Medical Center
Wednesday	Dec. 8	Dr. Nass, NYU Medical Center
Thursday	Dec. 9	Dr. Devinsky + EEG monitoring
Friday	Dec. 10	EEG monitoring
Saturday	Dec. 11	EEG monitoring
Monday	Dec. 13	Dr. Lombroso (AM) Dr. Holmes (PM)
Tuesday	Dec. 14	BEAM Test at Children's Hospital, Boston
Wednesday	Dec. 15	Dr. Volkmar
Thursday	Dec. 16	Dr. Volkmar
Friday	Dec. 17	Dr. Denison

Monday, November 1, 1993, 4:30 PM—Dr. Constantinou

Dr. Constantinou had instigated this appointment in an effort to convince us to cancel our trip to the United States. "I can tell you what they will say now," he said. "There will be three groups. Some will say that David has LKS, others Childhood Disintegrative Disorder, and others autism."

We were touched by his concern for our family's welfare.

Fred responded, "Dr. Constantinou, we wouldn't contemplate this trip if the expenses were in any way going to jeopardize our other children's futures or our subsequent lifestyle."

"What you are saying may well be true but I need to be able to look back on this segment of my life and feel that I tried my hardest for David," I added.

He respected our stand and offered his best wishes for our trip.

Wednesday, November 10, 1993

We met Dr. Jean Aicardi this afternoon at his friend Dr. Hopkins' surgery. This was the first time I had met a world-famous person and I was eager in my anticipation. Dr. Aicardi's demeanor and manner were humble, yet precise and conscientious. His conclusion regarding David disappointed us as he offered no suggested treatments or hope for improvement.

"The diagnosis of autistic regression is beyond doubt and there is no obvious brain lesion or biochemical disturbance to account for it."

That evening, when we returned home, a letter from Dr. Rosenbloom had arrived. "I enclose a rather depressing follow-up article to the one that you read and that was published in 1978." According to the longitudinal study, the prognosis for CDD children is bleak. All eight of the children were functioning at an intellectual level below the age at which they were first noticed to be regressing. "All of the boys masturbated openly during adolescence." The sentence felt as though it was wedged between the sides of my skull. I continued with the planning and routines of my life but whenever I paused, that ugly sentence flashed again in my brain. In summary, Dr. Rosenbloom described CDD as an acquired form of autism with an adverse developmental prognosis and unidentified etiology.

Although severely depressing in the short term, I felt relief and new strength. With knowledge, we could make management plans for David's future. Our four lives were not to be casualties of the emerging tragedy of David. At the same time, impetus grew for my continuing search for a cause of regression. Our son had the advantage of being born more than 20 years after Dr. Rosenbloom's children and new medical technology might eventually lead us to a more definitive diagnosis, treatment, and then an improvement or even a cure for David.

For David, a differential diagnosis was his only hope. It was as though our high-functioning, extroverted, and affectionate child was intact but locked away in a brain that had altered functioning. Maybe the process that had so insidiously occurred would never be identified. On the other hand, with identification, reversal, elimination, or even reduction of the abnormal process might not be possible. Within the context of my commitments to my marriage, children, and career, I would do my utmost to find out.

Wednesday, November 17, 1993
Today, we went to the travel agent to finalize the flight details of our impending trip. We decided to travel economy class and take along an adult to share the care of David. In addition, with a baby-sitter, Fred and I would have some fun along the way. We would ask Jenny Bolland to accompany us as she was outstanding in her management of David and pleasant company. When we were at appointments, Jenny could visit schools for autistic children and so broaden her expertise.

Friday, November 19, 1993, 3:30 PM—Chiropractor
A friend had told me of a chiropractor who specialized in treating children with learning disabilities. Her autistic son had improved noticeably while undergoing a course of manipulations. David appeared to enjoy his chiropractic sessions and I enjoyed hearing of selected successes of the practitioner with disabled children. Unfortunately, the discernible positive effects of the treatment ended here.

Friday, November 26, 1993
I was struck by a sudden realization. In a little more than a week, we were to pay more than U.S. $20,000 for 3 days of EEG monitoring. Currently, David was on a course of the anticonvulsant Vigabatrin in an endeavor to eliminate possible subclinical seizure activity. This activity was exactly what we were hoping the EEG would uncover! What irony. Here I was, trying to eliminate and discover simultaneously. Hastily, I composed a fax to Dr. Devinsky. His reply reassured me and I immediately altered David's treatment regime according to his instruction. On December 6, David was to have his last dose of Vigabatrin. The monitoring was not to commence until December 9.

Saturday, December 4, 1993
We arrived at JFK Airport. I felt wonderful. The trip had been comfortable and David was in good spirits.

Monday, December 6, 1993
We arrived at Dr. Kolodny's office at 8 AM. There were wide empty corridors along which David might run and we had brought a selection of his favorite toys. Two hours later, Dr. Kolodny called David's name. As with Dr. Aicardi, Dr. Kolodny presented as particularly thorough and conscientious. He mentioned the possibility of David's extended family contributing blood samples so that particular DNA sequences might be compared. Another suggestion worth pursuing was the testing of frozen fibroblast material.

In his report, Dr. Kolodny wrote of the possibility of a seizure disorder and suggested that trials of a variety of anticonvulsants might be worthwhile.

He continued: "If this approach proves fruitless, then we are left with the diagnosis of Childhood Disintegrative Disorder, also known as Heller's dementia."

In summary, he concluded, "I do not know of any metabolic or infectious basis for Heller's syndrome. Such children have less eye contact than what I saw with David and you have reported on his speaking in sentences, which is also somewhat against this diagnosis." This sounded encouraging. We might end up with a rosier diagnosis yet.

Tuesday, December 7, 1993
Dr. De Vivo suggested organizing a "STIR" sequence MRI, as these were known to be useful in caes of partial seizures, particularly those of temporal origin. With efficiency, he organized this on the spot for the next day. We were to return for a second consultation when the results were available.

That evening, we decided to dine at the hotel restaurant. Jenny, Fred, and I were eager to talk. Already, she had seen two schools and we had news relating to Dr. De Vivo and our travels around Manhattan. We were engrossed in conversation a second too long. In synchrony, the three of us looked across to David's chair. His knees were where his face had been only moments before. He was standing on his chair, holding his penis, and about to urinate on the carpet below. Just in time, I reached forward and grabbed him. The two elderly waiters who were servicing our table looked over in horror and then muttered to each other. Thankfully, our anticipated ejection never eventuated and we stayed to finish the meal.

Wednesday, December 8, 1993

In the morning we trekked to Columbia University Medical Center for David to undergo the MRI. The long-suffering David was sedated, though not anesthetized as he had been in Perth. Once the testing was completed, we whisked our sleeping child back to NYU for our appointment with Dr. Nass. It was regrettable that David slept throughout the entire consultation.

Dr. Nass had meticulously studied the detailed records and video that I had sent a few weeks before. She was quite confident that David had LKS. As we left, she gave me a copy of a published article she had written, detailing a $5\frac{1}{2}$-year old child with LKS and a strikingly similar history to David.

"He was the 7 pound product of an uncomplicated pregnancy and delivery. Motor milestones were mildly delayed (i.e., he walked at 18 months). At age 3 years, staring spells had been noted over several weeks but no EEG correlation had been obtained." This child was treated with valproate and 2 months after anticonvulsant initiation, his vocabulary was reported at 200 words with frequent use of short phrases. What inspiring reading it made! However, I wondered if Dr. Nass would have been as confident regarding the etiology of David's condition if she had observed him awake.

The MRI report awaited us when we returned to the hotel. There was some promise. The radiologist wrote, "There is apparent cortical thickening of the right temporal gyrus." We were not at all sure what that meant and so Fred rang Dr. De Vivo. The doctor considered that further MRI evaluation was warranted so that the nature of the cortical thickening, along with that of a focus of signal intensity in the left frontal region, might be explored further.

Another investigation that he suggested was a positron emission tomography (PET) scan. With this technique, the focal point of seizure is sometimes discerned by the exposure of unusual metabolic activity in the brain using radioactive substances. Dr. De Vivo offered to refer us to an imaging center at UCLA that specialized in such scans for children.

Thursday, December 9, 1993
At 8 AM we met with Dr. Devinsky and David was admitted to the hospital for 3 days of EEG monitoring. This we considered to be our foremost appointment. Dr. Devinsky quizzed us on David's history. I was surprised as it had all been documented in the dossier that I had sent some weeks before. He seemed totally unfamiliar with the details.

Friday, December 10, 1993
At the hospital all was well. David was content and had quickly adjusted to the severe restriction placed by the monitoring leads.

Saturday, December 11, 1993
Fred arrived back at our room at around 7:30 AM after his overnight session with David. He related that at Dr. Devinsky's late afternoon visit the doctor had reported that no seizure activity had been identified. For this reason, he had decided that David should be kept awake all that night and that the monitoring should continue until lunchtime on Sunday.
"He said it so casually," said Fred. "As though keeping David awake all night was as easy as blowing your nose."

Sunday, December 12, 1993
The results of the EEG study dashed our hopes of a definitive LKS diagnosis. Dr. Devinsky reported that sharp transients around the left midtemporal region were present but there was no clearly associated epileptogenic potential. Moreover, no focal abnormalities were observed. We were disappointed but had no regrets. Consultations with two Harvard professors of pediatric neurology and a return to New York for a second MRI at Columbia were among avenues of elucidation that remained open.

Monday, December 13, 1993

This morning was our appointment with Dr. Lombroso, a prominent child neurologist. After a routine physical examination of David, Dr. Lombroso expressed interest in the results of the 4 days of monitoring. We were to meet again on Friday afternoon when he would discuss the results of tomorrow's BEAM test, along with his overall impressions of David's condition.

Next was our appointment with Dr. Holmes. I surmised that he had probably acquired the Harvard Chair of Neurophysiology on the retirement of Dr. Lombroso. Dr. Holmes suspected that David had a variant of LKS. In his report, he wrote of David's aphasia as taking a waxing and waning course and considered that this factor and the temporal lobe discharges demonstrated in his EEGs provided some evidence. He suggested three treatments: steroids, gammaglobulin, and the anticonvulsant Felbamate. With regard to the problem of David's hyperactivity, Dr. Holmes suggested three different medications. The man's positivity encouraged me.

Over dinner that evening, Jenny described fragments of her visit to the Boston Higashi School. She told of the strong Japanese cultural presence and how all children were involved in activities. The student orchestra performed at the morning assembly and each child marched with the group. In addition, she was impressed by the fact that no child was allowed to opt out from his environment by self-stimulating.

Tuesday, December 14, 1993

Early this afternoon was David's BEAM test appointment. "Brain electrical activity mapping" is the full title of this test. It was explained to us as something akin to an EEG insofar as electrodes are used, but in addition visual and auditory evoked potentials are obtained.

Once again, the electrodes were fitted to David's head and, under the circumstances, his uncooperative behavior seemed totally reasonable. With wiring completed, I was guided to a chair in a darkened booth where with David on my knee, the entire testing session took place. David was subjected to the stimuli of speech, music, and light.

The BEAM report was gratifying in that the result was abnormal but unenlightening in that it did not add any insight to an etiology for David's regression. In their summary, Drs. Lagae and Duffy wrote: "Overall this study must be considered abnormal. Although no classic indications for an encephalopathic process or seizure disorder are detected, evidence for a global processing abnormality is indicated."

Wednesday, December 15, 1993
I was pleased to meet Dr. Volkmar this morning. His contribution in bringing CDD to the attention of pediatricians had been significant. In particular, he was largely responsible for the proposed listing of the disorder in the fourth edition of the *Diagnostic and Statistical Manual* scheduled to be published in May 1994.

Fred and I were eager to see two video clips of other patients. As with the video we had prepared of David, there was footage of each child, both before and after regression. The first was of a handsome, dark-haired boy. He was about 2½ years old and had been photographed on Christmas morning. Obligingly, he said hello and wished his absent grandparents a Happy Christmas. Dr. Volkmar then commented, "Note the 'big boy' underpants." The second segment showed the same child less than a year later. He had been photographed through the glass wall of Dr. Volkmar's playroom. It was tragic to see the same child in diapers and licking the glass.

Next we viewed a pale-faced, blond boy of about 2 years who was sitting in his highchair and singing *Happy Birthday.* After regression, he was pictured at school rolling on the floor and laughing to himself, oblivious to those around him. Later, he wantonly lunged at a shelf that supported a dozen or so books and caused the lot to fall to the floor. I almost cried for the parents. Yet to some degree, seeing these children on film was therapeutic. Dr. Volkmar kindly agreed to pass on my details to the parents of each of his CDD patients.

Thursday, December 16, 1993
Today David underwent his final evaluations with Dr. Volkmar's team. The written report that followed suggested no treatments other

than behavioral intervention but confirmed our belief that the diagnosis of CDD applied to David.

We then headed back to New York and Columbia Presbyterian Medical Center for David's second brain imaging. This second imaging cleared the two uncertainties that had been raised by the first. The suspected cortical thickening was found to be overlapping folds of tissue. The area of signal intensity in the left frontal region was deduced to be a tiny heterotopic focus rather than an angioma. Both irregularities were described as normal variants.

Friday, December 17, 1993

This morning's appointment with Dr. Denison did not add much to our understanding or management of David's problem. She wrote that his problem suggested global and pervasive processing difficulties affecting both social and cognitive development.

This afternoon we were again in Dr. Lombroso's reception area. I was very keen to learn of his overview. Dr. Lombroso recalled how David's dossier had led him to suspect that David was a likely candidate for an LKS diagnosis. Now, he had decided that David's problem was global rather than aphasic. This position was supported by the results of the BEAM test, which he considered to suggest degrees of dysfunction to several brain areas but with no evidence of a seizure disorder. He finished with suggestions for various symptomatic treatments for David's psychosis and overactivity.

Saturday, December 18, 1993

Fred had pursued Dr. De Vivo's referral to the Ahmanson Biochemical Imaging Center at UCLA so that David might have a PET scan. David's appointment was for the following Tuesday.

Monday, December 20, 1993

Now it was David's time for fun. We journeyed to Disneyland. David sat contentedly for three turns in a large green cup from "Alice In Wonderland" and almost seemed mesmerized by the rotational and rocking movements and the accompanying music. While still in Fantasyland, Donald Duck approached, whereupon David promptly bit his tail!

Tuesday, December 21, 1993
     With optimism, we arrived for the PET scan. Here was one last chance for a nonsymptomatic diagnosis. Fred and I sat and viewed a monitoring screen as the now sedated David underwent his scan. We watched enthralled by the colorful cross-sectional images of his brain. "Each color represents the metabolism of a different substance," explained the operator. "Basically, we are looking for an asymmetry of metabolism," he finished.
     I was grateful for the explanation as now I could contemplate the changing images with more purpose. "This looks promising," said Fred as he pointed to an obvious asymmetry on the monitor. The kaleidoscopic picture before us continually changed with respect to both shape and orientation of color. On a number of occasions, we commented to each other on slight asymmetries. We left full of hope.
     A few hours later we were back on campus, eager to hear the report of the testing.
     "The results were normal," Dr. Schnider reported.
     This was one of the lower points of my life.
     "But we observed asymmetries during the scanning," I said.
     "The asymmetries you saw must have been artifacts," he replied.
     "Why are you pursuing a Landau–Kleffner diagnosis when David has had no seizure? LKS is a seizure disorder. So what you are doing doesn't make sense. Your son is autistic and I suggest that you treat the symptoms behaviorally."
     His words hit my head like rocks and the lower moment in my life descended still further. There was no point in responding to this man's question and comments. The consultation ended and with a determined effort, I smiled and thanked him as we left.
     "He thinks he knows it all," I said to Fred.
     "He thinks he knows more than the world experts on David's condition. The man's an arrogant idiot."
     "He's supposed to be a specialist in epilepsy and he doesn't even know that a third of children with LKS have only subclinical seizures."

"He doesn't even realize that autism is a collection of symptoms and an umbrella term for a number of conditions."

Fred was now tired of my emotional monologue and, with a piercing stare of his blue eyes, said authoritatively, "Maybe he's right. David doesn't have LKS."

I was silenced and tried to focus on something more pleasurable in my life. Food, wine, and dinner tonight were manifest strongly in my mind.

"Tonight will be our last meal in America. Let's go to the pizza restaurant we noticed a few streets away," I said.

"Okay, but let's get a taxi driver to show us Beverly Hills first," said Fred.

Thursday, December 23, 1993

The 19-hour flight from Los Angeles to Sydney was therapeutic in that I had the opportunity to muse over my experiences of the last 3 weeks. Did I consider that the trip had been successful? Did we get value for the money we had spent?"

Obviously, we had not achieved our most sublime hope of a treatable and curable diagnosis for David. Next on our lists of aims was simply an etiology for David's condition. This too had eluded us. It did not take long to deal with the negatives. Now, I moved to the positives:

☐ David is listed as a patient of some of the world's foremost pediatric neurologists. I would contact them periodically to ask of developments.

☐ Our concerns that David had a progressive disorder were largely put to rest.

☐ Testing had been completed that we had been unable to organize in Australia. Extended video EEG monitoring, BEAM testing, and PET scanning had all been performed.

☐ More sensitive MRI techniques not available in Australia had confirmed that the tiny spot on the left frontal region of David's brain was heterotopic matter rather than an angioma.

☐ Treatments had been suggested and we would now work systematically through them.

☐ We had viewed videos of children who presented similarly to David. It felt better to know there were other parents who had suffered comparable tragedies and were experiencing similar ongoing problems.

☐ Dr. Volkmar had agreed to pass on our details to the parents of other CDD children.

☐ It had been an enlightening and inspiring experience to meet world experts in their field. I was impressed by their compassion and humility.

My doubts as to the accomplishments of our extravagant jaunt had now vanished.

Friday, January 14, 1994

David had always enjoyed being immersed in water and now he was to have three lessons a week in our home pool. His teacher, Richard, was tireless, patient, and dedicated to our cause of teaching David to become mobile in our pool. At present, his enjoyment was restricted because in all areas the water was out of his depth. This left the options of watching David cling to the edge, play on the steps, or supporting and playing with him in the water.

Saturday, January 29, 1994

For the first time, I spoke with another CDD parent! Stephen Ferris of Canberra telephoned. He is the father of $3^1/_2$-year-old Laura who had begun regressing at the age of about 27 months. The onset of the regression coincided with a vaccination of Prohibit, which is used to provide protection against meningitis. This was reminiscent of David's case where I had originally considered his May immunization with the vaccine to have been a precipitating factor in his insidious decline, which was first noticed a few months later.

It was invigorating to speak with this thoughtful, quietly spoken man. He too was making a concerted effort to find a cause and treatment for his daughter's acquired autism. Our conversation ended with a mutual agreement to exchange histories of our children and to forward new leads that might facilitate an increased understanding of the neurological illness that had invaded our lives.

The CDD Network had formed.

Monday, January 31, 1994

I picked up a Ritalin prescription from the hospital. Today, we were to begin treating David's hyperactivity. The effect of the Ritalin on David's behavior was amazing. He became quiet, attentive, and no longer bolted. "I can't quite grasp why no doctor prescribed this drug before," I said to David's program assistant after she had commented on David's improved performance in his series of Lovaas-type tasks.

Over the following month, my understanding of the Ritalin issue deepened. I had been quick to appreciate the desirable effects but now the downside was evolving. To a large degree, David's appetite had diminished and since the commencement of treatment, he had lost weight. He now looked skinny and undernourished.

The second side effect was just as intolerable. With considerable regularity, David had begun having aggressive outbursts at about three o'clock in the afternoon. This was new behavior for our previously happy and gentle child. Program assistants were regularly reporting that David had bitten them or tantrumed.

Our daily survival was threatened by the apparent impact on David's sleeping habits. Each evening at bedtime, David would exhibit a surge of overactivity. Sometimes, he would still be jumping vigorously on his bed at midnight. "It's as though the hyperactivity which is suppressed during the day is stored up and vented at night," commented Fred. The choice was easy. We discontinued the Ritalin.

A depression had slowly pervaded my outlook and I stopped worrying about death. Life seemed close to impossible and should my life have been taken, I would not have complained too loudly. It surprised me, but never did I consider suicide. My commitments to Fred, Tom, and Sarah, along with my underlying love of life and its opportunities for challenge and achievement may have been the reasons.

My response to a challenge usually consisted of a determined, organized, and sometimes lengthy effort. If unsuccessful, I would review my efforts and if it were plausible, modify my approach and try again. On occasions, I was left with no ideas for a change of approach. Then I would either alter or discard the challenge. At present, I wanted to drop the apparently impossible challenge of bringing up a child who was impossible to control without constant one-on-one supervision, a child who showed little affection or even acknowledgment of me as a mother, a child who, despite our best efforts at behavioral therapy, continued to regress. The huge management problems associated with David's illness had knocked me over and it seemed as though I couldn't get up. This new style of parenthood where the responsibilities are grossly magnified and extend through old age to death, coupled with a removal of the joys, did not suit me.

Tuesday, February 1, 1994, 9 AM—Dr. Parry
In an endeavor to document David's development, Dr. Parry had agreed to administer six monthly Griffith's Tests. Today, David's underwent his third testing. The results supported my observation of continued regression in the Hearing and Speech area. When first tested in October 1992, David's functioning in this area had been estimated to be 31.5 months, and 6 months later it had been 22 months. Today, his performance was rated as only 20.5 months.

Tuesday, February 15, 1994
I was grateful and relieved when my inner strength resurged. Our plans for our flat over the garage were ready for council approval. As I perused them with the architect, it felt as though I was beginning to regain control of my life. "By the end of the year our helper will have moved into our backyard respite facility," I anticipated with pleasure.

Sunday, February 20, 1994
We decided to celebrate David's fifth birthday a week early. His cake was the shape of a fat green caterpillar, complete with licorice legs. My choice was made because of David's persisting love of the book *Very Hungry Caterpillar.* He was certainly entranced but whether or not this was because of an association or a hope to grab for a taste of icing, I am not sure.

Monday, February 21, 1994

David could now swim the entire length of the pool. He had developed his own version of the dog paddle and sometimes he would even use it to swim underwater.

Regularly, I would swim with David and while in the water together it felt as though a major portion of David's disability had left him. Together we would play a game the two of us had developed. It was called "Ready, steady, go" and David would swim to me and I would hold him against my body with both arms. Here David would sit expectantly for half a minute or so, looking up at me with a huge grin. Then he would carefully recite the key words, usually with clear articulation.

"Ready, steady, go."

On hearing these words, I would throw him up into the air so that he would land on the water with a splash.

Wednesday, February 23, 1994, 9 AM—Dr. Batten

Dr. Batten was a general practitioner who specialized in naturopathic treatments for cancer and environmentally induced illnesses. A friend had mentioned that lead poisoning may cause intellectual regression. On explaining that David's serum lead was in the lower end of the normal range, she responded with: "Some doctors consider that lead levels in the hair are a more reliable measure as these are subject to less fluctuation."

I was not entirely convinced; especially when David's neurologist had said that he considered such analyses to be unreliable. But I decided to pursue the matter in any case.

As requested, Dr. Batten agreed to organize a hair analysis for David and I left with instructions for collection and forms to accompany a sample to a laboratory in Chicago.

The results were staggering. Within the classification of nutrient minerals, David's hair had recorded levels more than two standard deviations outside the mean for zinc, copper, sodium, and potassium. The concentrations of toxic minerals, lead, and aluminum were measured to be almost two standard deviations above the mean. I remembered a comment by Dr. Walsh as to the inaccuracy of hair analysis. Logically, I decided to have David's hair retested at an independent laboratory and compare the two sets of results. I sent a sample to a center in New South

Wales. The results supported Dr. Walsh's view and depleted any confidence I had in this form of testing. All of the nutrient minerals that had previously scored levels outside the normal range were now measured as being close to the mean. With reference to the toxic metals, lead was actually recorded as below the mean and aluminum only slightly above.

Visions came to me of a laboratory assistant in a white coat, working at a bench inside a suburban garage. On the computer monitor facing her was the facsimile of an Analysis Report Form and she was holding an electronic random number generator. Stacked to her right were a pile and a heap. The pile consisted of $50 checks ripe for banking while the heap was of sealed plastic bags that were labeled with patient details and contained hair samples. The procedure was simple. Details were typed into the computer from the plastic bags, which were then discarded unopened into the wastepaper basket. The recorded levels of the minerals were created using the random number generator and then typed into the computer. Printing and posting completed the process.

Friday, February 25, 1994
There were rewards today when I went to the mailbox. I opened the letter with the New York postmark first.

"We received your name and address from Dr. Volkmar as parents who would like to correspond with other parents in order to share information," began the letter.

I continued reading with excitement.

"Our other three children are fine, thank goodness, but as I'm sure you know it is heartbreaking to see your beautiful, normal-looking child act like an animal at times and always seeming to be out of it in terms of reality."

Empathy came easily as I thought of David trying to drink from a toilet while in New York.

"In public places, people don't understand, and give the parents mean looks and comments!"

Memories of David stealing hot chips from the plate of a horrified woman at a local food hall rushed to my mind.

"We want to wish the best to you and your child and really hope you can write to us!"

"Take Care, Madeline and Bob Catalano," concluded the letter. What a great opportunity I thought as I simultaneously thanked Dr. Volkmar for keeping his word. The second item of interest was a letter from New Zealand.

"Our son Nicky, now 8 years old, began slowly deteriorating about 4 years ago. He has been pretty stable for the last 2 years, but he has made very few advances, he just becomes a larger and larger 2-year-old."

The letter was signed, "Sheila Brown."

Once inside, I mused over an enclosure within the Catalanos' letter. It was entitled "Welcome to Holland" and had been written by the mother of a Down syndrome child. It didn't quite fit our situation as the parents of CDD children. For one reason, Down syndrome is apparent soon after birth. For another, the parents of such children do not need to search for a diagnosis, etiology, and treatment. In addition, the parents of Down children do not suffer the trauma of seeing their child's development disintegrate and then stagnate. And finally, Down children are usually sociable, loving, and verbal.

I decided to write an adaptation of "Welcome to Holland." Metaphor is often an aid to facing and coming to understand one's feelings. The article compared planning and giving birth to a child to the experience of planning and successfully executing a vacation to Italy. Giving birth to a Down syndrome child was likened to planning a trip to Italy and ending up in Holland.

My version told of a couple planning their Italian vacation, arriving and having a wonderful time at all of the regular tourist attractions. Then slowly or maybe suddenly, the scenario changed. The tourist maps didn't seem to be accurate, extracts from the phrase book were no longer understood, and at St. Michael's Square, the canals and gondolas had disappeared from Venice. The couple examined their environment more closely and studied and applied their phrase book more diligently, but to no avail. They even went to the central Tourist Bureau in Rome in an endeavor to clarify their problems.

"You're not in Rome," said the chief consultant. "You're in Amsterdam."

The couple were stunned by the man's lack of compassion and amazed at his statement. "How can Italy suddenly become Holland?" asked the wife.

"I don't think that you were ever in Italy," replied the expert.

"But we have photos of us both in front of the Leaning Tower of Pisa," said the husband in shocked disbelief.

I loved the allegory but the big problem of its application to CDD was the fact that Holland is just as attractive to tourists as Italy. Yet it is obviously ridiculous to try to pretend that having a child with CDD is on a par with parenting a normal child.

Sheila wrote very aptly, "I really liked the little tale about Italy and Holland, but I actually think Sierra Leone or some such country would have been a more appropriate choice than Holland!"

Monday, April 4, 1994

I had arranged to view the Education Support Unit for intellectually handicapped children at Loreto, the local Catholic primary school, with a view to a placement for David in 1995. The most startling factor for me was the high level of functioning of all 10 of the children compared to David. On my arrival, the teacher introduced me to the children, who immediately greeted me with considerable interest and enthusiasm. The children then continued with their work and I wandered through the classroom, observing and chatting to them as they drew pictures or wrote words to tell of their activities on the recent weekend.

Fifteen years before, I had enjoyed the experience of teaching mathematics to a class where the ability level was at the top of the subnormal scale. My lack of experience with the lower ability levels left me astounded with the children's inability to use patterns as a tool for generalizations. At the time, I was unable to appreciate the fact that some children, in particular my still-to-be-conceived son, were never even likely to arrive at the stage of perceiving the existence of a problem or indeed even understanding the concept of a problem. By comparison, failure to grasp an underlying pattern or strategy related to problem solving is indeed a tiny deficit.

Sunday, April 24, 1994

By now, I was in regular contact with Madeline Catalano, Sheila Brown, and Stephen Ferris and all four of us were keen to create a more formal network. Besides the considerable therapeutic benefits and opportunities for international friendships, I recognized the advantages of sharing any enlightening information that individual families gleaned pertaining to CDD. I formulated four aims for our network:

- ☐ To share information relating to CDD
- ☐ To provide support and encouragement to other families
- ☐ To increase the network so that there will exist a larger group of children whose case histories may assist researchers with an interest in CDD
- ☐ To inform appropriate persons of the existence of the network

I was surprised that the others had no suggestions to modify the aims. Pleasingly, this hastened our next endeavor, which was to recruit other parents of CDD children. Autistic associations and pediatricians were an obvious starting point. Over the next 6 months, our aims, along with the criteria for CDD and contact details, were published in a variety of periodicals and sent to a number of pediatricians.

Intermittently, one of us received an inquiry. Madeline had a letter requesting contact with similar parents placed in the *Advocate,* the quarterly newsletter of the Autism Society of America. Despite the wide circulation, she had only one inquiry, and this was from one of the two families who had appeared on Dr. Volkmar's video.

"What a rare disorder CDD must be for us to come up with the same child from two quite independent sources," I wrote to Madeline. On second consideration, I remembered Dr. Volkmar's suggestion that the condition may not be as rare as first thought.

"It is indeed likely that many, if not most, cases of CDD have mistakenly been diagnosed as autism in recent years."

A fax from a father in Florida indicated that news of our network was reaching a desirable audience. "We received your name from a seminar in Chicago on autism. We believe our 4-year-old son fits the description of CDD. We also feel he was afflicted at the age of 2 due to him receiving routine immunizations (hepatitis B). . . ."

Monday, May 2, 1994—Dr. Loh, Immunology Clinic
I had chosen to consult with Dr. Loh, Perth's only pediatric immunologist, as a number of doctors had suggested that David's autism

might have an immunological basis. Immunological testing revealed nothing apart from slightly raised levels of immunoglobulin E. Dr. Loh placed no significance on this result but agreed to consider a trial of intravenous gammaglobulin as suggested by a number of the eminent neurologists who had reviewed David's case. Next on my list, though, was the treatment with corticosteroids.

Tuesday, May 3, 1994, 3:30 PM—Horseback riding
For the past year, David had enjoyed weekly horseback riding lessons at the Claremont Therapeutic Riding Centre. This organization specialized in providing riding experiences for disabled people. While on horseback David would be asked to follow simple instructions. For example, his teacher would hand him a can and say, "Put this on the red stick." The assistant would then lead the horse to a group of three or four different colored poles. Here, David was required to make his choice and then place the can over the appropriate stick. As with most things, the accuracy of his response varied from week to week. David's savored time during the lesson was trotting. The second the instructor permitted the horse to break into a trot, David's expression would change from contented to ecstatic.

Thursday, May 5, 1994
The previous December, Dr. Lombroso had suggested testing David's biotinidase levels. Today, David underwent a blood test and a frozen sample of David's platelets was to be sent to Auckland, which was the closest center providing this specialized test. Results later confirmed that David had normal levels of this enzyme.

Thursday, May 19, 1994, 8:15 AM—Interview with Geoff Matthews
Today was David's interview at Christ Church Grammar School, which we hoped was to confirm his admittance into the preparatory school the following year. "How about a tablet of Ritalin at 7:30?" I said to Fred as I rummaged through the top shelf of the pantry trying to locate the discarded medication. The three of us presented for the interview promptly and David was a silent, placid angel. The principal

and the teacher in the Education Support Unit agreed to accept David's enrollment. Their only doubts related to our insistence at providing a full-time aide as they considered that this might not be warranted. "What a coup!" I exclaimed to Fred with happiness as we walked to the car.

Thursday, May 26, 1994, 4 PM—Dr. Walsh
    We met with Dr. Walsh who purported that if David's syndrome was LKS or a related disorder, there was a 50% chance of a cure with the steroid treatment. "It's certainly a longshot," said Fred.
    "Yes, but the unpleasant side effects are reversible so I think we should give him the opportunity," I replied.

Wednesday, June 1, 1994
    At 8 AM a visiting nurse from Princess Margaret Hospital arrived to administer David's first injection of prednisolone, a synthetic corticosteroid hormone. This trial was to begin with large doses and gradually taper over the final stages of a 6-month period.

Wednesday, June 8, 1994, 9 AM—Dr. Parry
    It was only 4 months since the last Griffith's Test, so testing was less formal today. David performed surprisingly well to Dr. Parry's requests, and his report mentioned the improved quality of David's progress. I would have loved to have shared this enthusiasm. On the contrary, I considered that most areas of David's development had stagnated and that his expressive language skills had actually declined.

Friday, June 24, 1994, 8:30 AM—Reyne to play
    During 1994, David attended the local kindergarten four mornings a week. His inclusion was achieved with the help of his full-time aide, Elsa. Another 5-year-old, Reyne, had taken a special interest in helping and befriending David. On Fridays, there was no kindergarten and at Reyne's request, I had organized with his mother for him to visit. Elsa

had carefully chosen a series of tasks from David's intervention program that were particularly amenable to either sharing or turn-taking. It was heartening to see David's response to Reyne. He greeted him with a wide smile and repeated his name clearly. The first activity in Elsa's agenda was playing "Thomas the Tank Engine." This game involved a player rotating a spinner and then, if successful, adding an engine shape to an allocated space on his board.

David completed his turn with some prompts from Elsa. Looking across to Reyne, he beamed as if to indicate that it was now his turn. "At least, his social skills seem to have stopped regressing," I thought with relief.

Monday, June 27, 1994, 12:30 PM—Tony Schneider

The Young Autism Project was a research project that was attempting to replicate the work of Lovaas at the University of California, Los Angeles. David was included in this study and Tony Schneider was a psychologist employed by the university to monitor David's progress. His testing ranked David's receptive language as 12 months and expressive as 15 months. These results reflected my own informal assessment of David's language.

Thursday, June 30, 1994, 4 PM—Dr. Walsh

While on the steroids, David's physical condition was to be monitored monthly by Dr. Walsh. Apart from excessive weight gain, bloatedness, and hypotonia, the treatment temporarily reduced bone density and, rarely, liver malfunction was induced. After only 4 weeks of treatment, changes in David's body were observable. His weight had climbed from 20 kg to 22. Instead of lean, he now looked thick-set. I was not concerned about the weight gain as I understood this to be inevitable, but of considerable concern was David's articulation. Since the commencement of treatment, his verbalizations had become increasingly slurred and his lips seemed not to move when he spoke. In addition, his spontaneous speech was now almost nonexistent. Maybe the change in speech represented the evolution of David's mysterious disorder. Certainly, Dr. Walsh had not heard of any similar response to steroid therapy.

Monday, July 4, 1994

Sarah skipped in happily from the letter box and announced with gusto, "There's a parcel from New Zealand, Mummy." Letters from fellow networker Sheila were always received enthusiastically by us both. From Sarah's point of view, there was usually an enclosure from Sheila's daughter, Katie, who was now her pen pal. From my point of view, Sheila's positive and practical approach to the handling of her nearly 9-year-old son, along with her well-chosen appendixes, were always uplifting as well as informative. One enclosure particularly caught my attention. It was a copy of a newscutting from *The Star*, an Irish daily paper, and the headline was "How David was cured by a miracle: Save others from my son's hell." I read on.

"Mrs. Kath Howard's young son was a mindless uncontrollable demon until a miracle cure was found for his illness. Now she wants the Government to encourage research into the cause of his complaint, disintegrative psychosis." The article continued to describe how David deteriorated at about 18 months around the time of a measles vaccination. Two years later his parents consulted Dr. Keith Mumby, an allergy expert from Manchester. Dr. Mumby performed a series of tests and concluded that David had 22 allergies, mainly from dairy foods. His next step was to develop antidotes to help his patient develop resistance to them.

Within weeks there was a noticeable improvement and $3^1/_2$-year-old David Howard began to talk for the first time, play like a normal child, and show affection for his brothers and sisters. Needless to say, I found the article inspiring reading, particularly as the exceedingly rare diagnosis of disintegrative psychosis (CDD) had been cited as the condition originally affecting Dr. Mumby's patient. I faxed Keith Mumby and was delighted to receive his reply within the day. He wrote, "I suggest we proceed to a fairly drastic diet I call the 'eight foods diet.' The idea is to eliminate all normal foods, but without the severity of a fast. The patient eats only exotic foods by which I mean foods he doesn't normally eat."

I read on to learn that the diet was comprised of two vegetables, two fruits, two meats, and two grains, all of which had been eaten at most infrequently. The closing paragraph mentioned other possible treatments and closed with: "ONE THING AT A TIME is the golden rule." I filed the information for later reference.

Thursday, August 11, 1994
David had his first session of sensory integration therapy today with the occupational therapist, Vicki Hawley. The consultation room clearly met David's approval. It was furnished with children's gym and play apparatus. To the right was a long wooden ramp that ended with a platform next to a pile of tractor tubes. David lay on his stomach on a scooter board at the lower end of the wooden ramp. With Vicki's help he pulled himself up the incline by clasping his hands to the low sides and pulling the wheeled board forward. Finally, his efforts enabled him to roll himself onto the horizontal section at the upper end.

With a swift movement, Vicki turned the scooter board around so that David, still lying face down, was looking down the ramp.

"Say 'ready, go,' David," said Vicki.

"Ready steady go," said David in a quiet, muffled voice that only Vicki could hear.

She released her hold with a push and down the ramp he quickly rolled.

Tuesday, August 23, 1994, 2 PM—EEG
Again David was sleep-deprived in preparation for his EEG the following day. Awake to midnight and then up again at 5 o'clock was the now-familiar routine. This time one of David's program assistants would ensure the implementation.

Our endeavor to maintain our lifestyle as David's mental condition deteriorated had resulted in a gradual increase in the hours of hired help in our home. On weekdays, an assistant for David arrived at 6:45 AM and finished at the kindergarten 2 hours later when he was placed in Elsa's care. In the afternoons and evenings, another assistant would be David's shadow until half past seven.

As a consequence, life was now less stressful than it had been for more than 2 years. Internal and external doors were able to remain unlocked as I no longer had to contain David in the same room. I could answer the telephone without dropping it in a panic as David came into view with a fistful of margarine. The nightmare of cooking dinner and endeavoring to supervise the overactive David was only a memory. During the meal, the assistant sat next to David. His habit of eating a mouthful, jumping up, and running around the family area was severely checked. Only once or twice a meal would he now manage to make a complete break away from his minder.

In the past, I knew that successful completion of my simultaneous tasks was impossible. Many times, after an hour of cooking and serving, punctuated by chasing and rescuing David from his mess-making escapades, or attempted bolts through an overlooked, unlocked door, I would be reduced to a crying, screaming mess.

Reports from the literature of 90% of CDD children ending in residential care made sense. David the child was to stay with his family. Fred and I considered that the huge increase in our household expenditure was well spent.

Thursday, August 25, 1994, 5:30 PM—Dr. Walsh

At this appointment with Dr. Walsh I learned that David's EEG was normal—a pity as I never quite gave up hoping that a highly treatable abnormality would emerge. Or failing this, there still remained the hope that I might learn of the process that had caused his regression and halted his further development.

Since our last consultation David's speech had disappeared altogether and for a few weeks he was heavy, bloated, and mute. Then came the noise. Gradually, he began making nonverbal vocalizations that could most accurately be described as "bops and beeps."

David's voracious appetite, along with the fluid retention caused by the hormones, meant that he was now an overweight 26 kg. Unexpected side effects had also reared. His beautiful blond hair had darkened and had the smell and greasy appearance associated with adolescence. Fine downy hair had grown on his genital area and upper back.

"I want to see the treatment through," I said to Fred.

"It's hard to watch our poor boy lose his body along with his mind; but apparently noticeable improvement doesn't usually come until after 3 months."

Tuesday, October 18, 1994, 1 PM—S.I.T.

David had remained a client of Vicki's, and today was a weekly sensory integration therapy session. She had observed the disappearance of the residual of David's speech. Whereas initially he could manage,

"Ready, steady, go" at the top end of the scooter board ramp, now he could seldom say even the first syllable.

Happily, the disappointing decline of David's expressive language had been accompanied by a corresponding improvement in his receptive skills. "You've dropped a piece," I said to David as he was carrying a wooden puzzle from shelf to table. Within seconds, I was expecting to move to his side to physically prompt him to go back and pick up the puzzle piece. My mouth opened in amazement. On hearing my comment, David had stooped, picked up the errant piece, and continued with the task. Some hours later, he had darted off as I was washing his face. "Come back, David," I instructed firmly. He came back! I was jubilant. This was the first positive change I had noted since the beginning of the regression.

Thursday, December 1, 1994—Conclusion of steroid trial

Today, David had his final injection and the corollary was lengthy. No more visiting nurses invading our sanctuary at 8 AM each morning. No more was David to be subject to daily intramuscular injections in his deeply bruised buttocks. The steroid trial had ended with David weighing in at an obese and bloated 30 kg—a 50% weight gain. I felt cruel, knowing that it was Fred's and my decision that had caused these massive physical changes. The emergence of frequent meaningless vocalizations, the decline in expressive language, and the resurgence of some receptive skills were concurrent with the trial. Whether the overlap was coincidental or related I would never know.

Tuesday, December 6, 1994

Our flat on top of the garage was finished. The builders had completed their contract and now I had the pleasurable task of choosing the furnishings. It was a quiet haven, untainted by the bustle that almost constantly permeated our house. "I could retire here," I thought.

Wednesday, December 7, 1994

With the steroid trial behind us, I met with Dr. Loh to ask him to organize the intravenous gammaglobulin treatment for David. He indicated his willingness to arrange and supervise six three-weekly infusions but was careful to stress the risks. Overseas there had been reports of hepatitis C contamination and more generally severe allergic reactions, fevers, and vomiting had been documented. We were not unnerved. The major complications were exceedingly rare and we were anxious to try the suggested treatments resulting from our U.S. and eastern Australian tours. For $2^1/_2$ years, we had watched the regression and stagnation of David's development. Consequently, any definite improvement, however slight, would have been gratefully received.

Monday, January 23, 1995
Parma moved into the flat. My idea of a backyard respite facility had germinated 18 months before and today it had come to fruition. Fred and I had met Parma about a year earlier when she had joined David's intervention program as an assistant. She was quiet, patient, reliable, and dedicated to doing her best for David. In my choice, "quiet" had been an essential criterion. I certainly didn't want to employ a raging extrovert who might bring to our property a stream of noisy visitors.

Tuesday, January 24, 1995, 9 AM—Dr. O'Leary
Today a blood sample was to be drawn from David. Via Sheila Brown, I had learned of continuing research at the University of Birmingham by Dr. Rosemary Waring into a phenolsulfotransferase deficiency. An article reported that all 14 children tested with induced autism had exhibited low levels of the enzyme. Inquiries by Dr. O'Leary, a clinical biochemist at Princess Margaret Hospital, revealed that it was considerably cheaper to send frozen platelets to Britain than to set up the required assay in Perth. Kindly, he agreed to organize the collection and preparation of the specimen for transportation. David's sample was collected with only minor protests.

"Your turn now," said the assistant looking across to Dr. O'Leary who had now reentered the room and was rolling up his sleeve. "Just providing a control," said the biochemist, obviously responding to my puzzled expression.

"I'd be happy to do that," I said, feeling guilty that this stranger was donating his blood for the benefit of my son.

"No, best if I do. I'm unrelated," replied the scientist.

Monday, January 30, 1995, 8:15 AM—Infusion at PMH

Dr. Loh had organized for David to undergo six immunoglobulin infusions. The first was scheduled for today. Again, David's high level of tolerance of restrictive treatments amazed me. The insertion of the drip met with physical resistance but, this completed, my overactive David was happy to sit in a chair and watch television, blindly play with a hand-held electronic device, or rummage through books with the occasional tasting of a page.

Late in the afternoon, the removal of the intravenous attachment from David's arm seemed to him a signal to be overactive again. Within seconds, he had jumped from the chair and made a dash for the door. I immediately thought of Sarah's question of almost a year before: "What would you do if David was only pretending to be sick?" My answer had been, "Give a party." I wondered if David had more control over his behavior than any of us realized.

Saturday, February 18, 1995

I had begun a weight chart on December 1, immediately after David's last steroid injection. It was astounding that his weight loss had occurred as speedily as his weight gain. Correspondingly, David's appearance and energy level had revived. His corpulent, inflated appearance was now superseded by a slim and toned torso. The creamy complexion, blonde curls, and handsome features had returned.

Tuesday, February 28, 1995, 1:30–7 PM—Infusion

David's second infusion was today. Despite our close scrutiny, we had not yet perceived any change in his presentation.

Friday, March 3, 1995, 7:30 AM—AIT

Auditory integration training (AIT) is a hearing enhancement training process for the receptive sensory anomalies commonly associated with autism and a variety of other disorders. Using specially designed equipment, sound intensity is randomized. Audiological information may be used by the practitioner to enhance and filter frequencies. Along these lines, the Frenchman Guy Berard developed a modified musical program that was designed to be played through headphones to participants over ten 30-minute sessions.

AIT with the audiologist Felicia Schmaman began today. Over a 10-day period, David was booked to have 10 half-hour sessions of treatment. The sessions were relaxing and enjoyed by us both. David would sit on Felicia's sofa wearing earphones and playing with a selection of his favorite and most transportable toys. Through Felicia's association with schools for autistic children in Victoria, she mentioned that she knew of one or two children who might meet the criteria for CDD.

David's auditory training did not precipitate any discernible change in his behavior. The only attributable gains were my acquaintance with the knowledgeable Felicia and her willingness to distribute network information to prospective parents.

Monday, April 17, 1995—Leave for Yallingup

This was to be our first holiday with all five of us since our Malaysian Nightmare of '92. Along with two assistants, we planned a week at the seaside, tourist town of Yallingup. Parma was rostered to integrate David for 8 hours each day and Lisa the remaining 5 or 6 hours of his waking time. It worked well. Donned in wet suits, all five of us and assistant would cross the road to the beach each morning. David delighted in splashing in the shallows and being washed ashore by the occasional wave. We had discovered the recipe for David to rejoin our family. In retrospect, it was obvious but on a daily basis, we had always underplayed the impact of the management problems associated with David's illness. As a consequence, we had never employed the level of assistance needed.

Wednesday, April 26, 1995

Recently, David's name had moved to the top of the waiting list of Catholic Care, a welfare organization of the Catholic Church that provided services to the intellectually handicapped and their families. My first visit to the Respite House broadened my education in relation to human handicap. In a wheelchair, with four lifeless limbs and an expression indicating an obliviousness to her surroundings was 8-year-old Emma. She would certainly meet the criteria for autism but her diagnosis was cerebral palsy. Mute, autistic, incontinent, quadriplegic, intellectually retarded, and others—almost every symptomatic description of disability that came to mind fitted the unfortunate child whom I now greeted.

David's disabilities paled by comparison. I thought back to last year when I had visited the Educational Support Unit at Loreto where the low level of disability of the students seemed to magnify David's handicap.

Saturday, May 6, 1995

Tom was now in the seventh and final year of his primary education at the local primary school. In 1996, he would begin his secondary education at Christ Church. Today, he and other applicants sat for a broad academic exam and from these results and subsequent interviews of finalists, five scholarship winners would be chosen. I estimated that Tom had a fighting chance of success as he had scored at high distinction level in a national mathematics competition and his creative writings had increasingly astounded me with their high level of originality and entertainment value.

Tuesday, June 13, 1995

A secretary from Christ Church telephoned.

"Thomas did quite well in the scholarship examination. Mr. House wants to meet him."

Friday, June 16, 1995

Prior to his interview, Tom gathered together as many certificates and awards for his achievements as he could muster. When we arrived for Tom's interview, the deputy headmaster, Mr. House, beckoned us to enter. We talked of David who it seemed was known to all staff and students, even though the secondary section was run as a separate entity. Perhaps it was because he had been the first student of the school to swim a lap of the pool in full uniform. Peta, David's aide, was accompanying him from classroom to oval during the lunch break. The pool gate was open, and David had made an obvious decision. As soon as he saw the opportunity, he escaped from her care, ran to the pool, and immersed himself in its cool waters. Or maybe David was well known because he was easily the most disabled student ever to attend the school.

Wednesday, June 21, 1995

"I didn't get a scholarship, Mummy," Tom said.

"Don't worry. I still love you as much as ever. You did very well to get to interview stage," I answered, trying to sound supportive.

"Only kidding. I did, I did," he said excitedly. I thought of our second son whose development for 3 years had paralleled and at times even surpassed that of his older brother at the same age. Their lives were now moving in opposite directions.

Thursday, July 6, 1995

Six months previously, I had the pleasure of meeting Stephen Ferris, Laura's father who was traveling to Indonesia via Perth in relation to his job with the Department of Foreign Affairs in the national capital. Today, I met Sheila Brown, Nicholas's mother who was visiting her sister-in-law in Perth with her husband and two healthy children, Andrew and Katie.

Nicky had been accepted at a boarding school in New Zealand for handicapped children. The school was run according to the principles of Rudolph Steiner and apart from formal lessons in the classroom, each pupil was allocated jobs as part of a wider community. These jobs might be sweeping, picking fruit, washing dishes, and so on. Apart from staff and students, this community included disabled adults who had originally joined when children as students. Accommodation was in group homes that were each managed by group parents. It sounded wonderful. I was especially attracted by the fact that the system nurtured its students throughout their entire life.

Meeting Sheila was enlightening. This person had lived with CDD for 6 years. Not only had she survived the ongoing tragedy, but she was implementing a remedy that showed the promise of fulfilling both the family's and her son's long-term needs. Sarah and her pen pal, Katie, became friends in a more practical sense. Katie shared Sarah's room for the night and joined her at school for the day. A positive had evolved from David's illness!

Wednesday, July 26, 1995, 9 AM—Dr. Parry
We had another appointment with Dr. Parry. This time my observations concurred with his. He noted that David's receptive language appeared improved in that he could follow instructions more precisely. Expressive language, he acknowledged, had deteriorated from phrases to only occasional single words. The formal Griffith's Test yielded an estimate of 13.5 months in the area of Speech and Language.

Tuesday, August 8, 1995—Final infusion; review with Dr. Walsh
Throughout the year, no improvement had been noted in David. Since the steroid treatment he had remained close to mute. The noisy nonverbal vocalizations that first reared during this time had become a permanent part of his behavioral repertoire. On a positive note, the increased ability to follow single step instructions had remained.

Today was David's eighth infusion and there had been no observed change. Dr. Walsh arrived, and we agreed to discontinue the immunoglobulin trial. It was time to move on. Anticonvulsants as suggested by Drs. Deonna and Rapin were next on my list and I had prepared copies of their reports that mentioned these as appropriate treatments for David.

"I want to see an EEG before I decide which drug to prescribe," said Dr. Walsh.

"Meanwhile, I'll be able to try Dr. Mumby's Exotic Foods Diet," I thought.

"Are the results for the phenosulfotransferase deficiency back from the University of Birmingham?" I asked. I could still visualize the conscientious Dr. O'Leary preparing to donate his blood as a control for the test.

"Yes, David tested low and the control sample was within normal range," he replied.

"This is how metabolic disorders are discovered," he added.

A few days later a copied extract of the results arrived at home.

Of David's platelet analysis the report described: "We have isolated a crude preparation of the enzyme and have found that there is a different isoform from those usually seen."

I tried to contain my hope within reasoned limits. Research was in its early stages and as is often the case, lack of funds severely restricted the degree of progress.

Saturday, August 12, 1995

"I think it is now time to start the Eight Foods Diet," I wrote to Dr. Mumby of David Howard fame. With the help of David's live-in assistant, Parma, organization for the diet proceeded. We chose two exotic foods from each of four food groups:

Meat	Turkey, rabbit
Vegetables	Spinach, turnip
Fruit	Mango, kiwi
Carbohydrates	Rye, millet
Sea salt	
Bottled spring water	

For 14 days, David was to consume only listed items after which usual items from the family menu were to be gradually reintroduced. With his usual tolerance, David happily accepted his restricted fare. As there was no change, Dr. Mumby suggested we abandon the diet approach and consider a course of vitamin B_{12} injections.

Monday, September 11, 1995

Again, I had found it difficult to motivate myself for the sleep deprivation needed for David's EEG of 11 days ago. But discipline and David's assistants kept me moving forward according to schedule. I felt close to certain that the results would be uninformative, which proved to me again that I am no psychic.

Dr. Walsh read us the results, which described recurrent spike activity in the frontal regions. I remembered David's heterotopic spot in the left frontal region and an article by Dr. Thierry Deonna that I had read 2 years before. Again, I recalled his writing on Acquired Epileptic

Frontal Syndrome. The reference to Disintegrative Disorder was still foremost in my mind.

Of children with this epileptic disorder he wrote: "Many of the symptoms seen in our children resemble those found in the developmental disorders known as 'disintegrative psychosis.' . . . Frontal lobe syndrome could be one of the causes of this pattern of regression."

Now back to the present and to David's treatment with anticonvulsants. Dr. Walsh decided on a dual treatment beginning with carbamazepine and adding Vigabatrin to the regime 6 weeks later. Concern over David's ongoing loss of expressive skills provided a reason for another MRI of David's brain.

Sunday, January 21, 1996

At present, it is impossible to write a summary of my efforts with David. Three and a half years after onset is very much the beginning of the story.

I love David with the unconditional love of a parent and will always endeavor to protect and nurture him. Unless a successful treatment is found, my boy reached the pinnacle of his cognitive, social, and language development at age 3 years. For this reason, I am loathe to conclude my quest for a cure. I have a mental image of a path, along which I am traveling. Each treatment and test compares with the passing of a milestone. The monitoring of testing and treatment is essential. The invasive test that holds little promise of a useful result in terms of David's future must be bypassed. On the other hand, an obscure, noninvasive test such as that for the phenolsulfotransferase deficiency might provide future, if not immediate, insight into David's condition. The EEGs and the imagings of the brain are points of reference to which we will repeatedly return while David's disorder continues to evolve. They are inconvenient but have no side effects and might provide us with knowledge that can be utilized to improve David's prognosis.

Maybe I was the perfectionist chasing after a fragile type of happiness that depended on everything moving according to some inner plan. Things go wrong, nothing is more certain. "Maximizing the positives, minimizing the negatives, and eking out positives from negatives" might be an apt description for my revised inner philosophy.

A song that Tom brought home a few years ago is running like a circular tape in my head.

This is the song that never ends
It goes on and on my friend.
Some people started singing it
Not knowing what it was
And now they can't stop singing it forever just because
This is the song that never ends . . .

Like the song, David's development may always be trapped in the same short verse. If so, I will strive to optimize his enjoyment of the rendition.

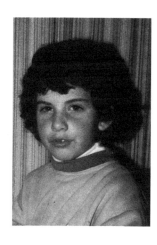

Six

Laura's Story

by Sue and Stephen Ferris

In this chapter, we describe how our bright little daughter, Laura, was cut off from the world by an "autistic regression"; how she has fared since; and our experience treating her.

We will comment on the treatments available for children with Childhood Disintegrative Disorder (CDD), and draw lessons from Laura's story. We believe intensive early intervention helped Laura. This should be made available to all children with CDD and other developmental disabilities, but requires early detection. Finally, we will briefly explore the causes of CDD, and suggest further research in this area.

To tell Laura's story, our language at times must be somewhat technical. Neither of us has a medical or psychological background, but since Laura's regression, we have devoted much energy attempting to understand her condition, and the tests and treatment for it. We hope our efforts to understand Laura's condition help others who care for a child with CDD. Therefore, we have included observations based on these efforts.

161

Laura's History

We live in Canberra, the capital city of Australia. We share the city with 300,000 others, who make up the vast majority of the population of the Australian Capital Territory, a small enclave in southeast Australia.

Laura was born on June 18, 1990, our second child. She was perfect, a very easy baby from the first day. We had to seek medical advice only for a facial rash that developed at 3 weeks of age (treated with antibiotics), and a bit later oral thrush and eczema. In the first 27 months, she achieved all of the "normal" milestones—smiled at 6 weeks, sat alone at 6 months, crawled at 8 months, and walked on her first birthday. She and her brother, Mark, who is 18 months older than Laura, always interacted very well. They enjoyed each other's company. For a while, Laura's speech was in many ways clearer than Mark's. For example, Laura said "Grandma" and "Granddad" from the age of about 18 months while Mark was still saying "Dada" and "Dadad." Laura used to love stories too. If we offered Mark a story, Laura would be the first one on our lap. "Postman Pat" was a favorite and, by the age of 2 years, she could recite whole paragraphs. She was familiar with all of the characters in these stories, and would point correctly to all of them when asked.

Laura also loved her little sister, Joanna, who was born in May 1992, a few weeks before Laura's second birthday. Joanna would only have to whimper and Laura would be there, giving her kisses and saying "Joanna, Joanna." There was absolutely no sign of the tragedy that was to strike in October 1992.

Our first indication that something was not quite right occurred when we started a home improvement project. We had been living in our house for about 18 months, and were finally starting to work on a driveway, with help from Laura's grandparents. Mark was showing all of the normal interest of an inquisitive 4-year-old. We left Laura in her room because she seemed tired and sleepy. She placidly stood in her bedroom, and sucked her pacifier. Occasionally she would look in a vague sort of way out of the window, but failed to respond to family members outside.

Soon Laura stopped welcoming her grandparents and uncle when they visited. She had always been very used to them, as they live only a short drive away. Laura always seemed to be busy, but it was not until later that we realized that her activity was aimless. She would often run about, or run backward and forward, but there was no purpose to all of the activity.

Another frightening occurrence was connected with the Postman Pat books. One day, while looking at her favorite book, she suddenly looked up, puzzled, and gave a little sob. It was obvious that she knew that she should be able to remember the story, but she could not. Tantrums started to creep into her daily life. She no longer found comfort in previously well-loved bedtime toys.

It is easy in hindsight for us to distinguish a number of incidents that could perhaps have alerted us sooner that we had the makings of a big problem. But at the time she still understood a number of instructions, and the normal requests made of any 2-year-old. She still had some speech and still sang songs. She could appear deaf at times, but so could Mark when we requested him to do something he did not want to do!

In mid-November 1992, Sue took Joanna for a routine 6-month checkup. While there Sue mentioned to the community nurse her concerns about Laura. The community nurse dismissed these, saying that Laura was a middle child and simply desired attention. We were not convinced, however, and resolved to spend extra time with her.

In early December 1992, we went on holiday to the coast, along with Laura's grandparents, uncle, and one of her uncle's friends. Laura thoroughly enjoyed the holiday, although she tantrumed for the first half-hour on arriving at the holiday units. All of the time, however, it was becoming clearer that something was wrong. She was not responding to us as the other children were. She appeared not to hear us much of the time, and was becoming locked in to her own little world where no one could reach her.

Tantrums were becoming more frequent, and shopping was becoming a nightmare. We would have to make sure Laura was in a pushchair, with a pacifier; and we would have to tip the pushchair back as we raced through the shop, to stop her digging her heels in and refusing to go farther.

Laura always had been very comfortable at her grandparents' house, but a visit a few weeks after the holidays seemed to unsettle her. For months afterward, Laura would only go into a small corner of the house. It was 6 months before she was comfortable again in the living area, and about 2 years before she would go upstairs again.

We finally decided to consult a general practitioner (GP) about Laura in January 1993. We had left Laura and the other children for a short time with their grandparents, so we could go shopping on our own. When we got back, there was chaos. Laura had slipped on the stairs and grazed her wrist. She went into hysterics. Her grandfather thought he would put on a Band-Aid—all children like Band-Aids! Not Laura! She refused to calm down until we got back.

In early February 1993, Laura was examined by the GP. He seemed quite concerned, but clearly had little comprehension of what we were saying. Most of the consultation was spent with the GP checking Laura's ears, throat, chest, and other areas, despite our telling him it was not that type of problem. However, he did refer Laura to a pediatrician.

Laura was examined by the pediatrician 2 weeks later. We were told it was definitely not normal for a child to lose all of her previously acquired skills. We remember him also asking if she would obey simple commands such as fetching a toy from her room. It was then that it became painfully obvious that we could not see her doing anything like that now. We had not wanted to acknowledge or accept how bad things had become.

Tests were arranged for Laura 2 days later at the local hospital. Urine tests, blood tests, a CAT scan, and an EEG were ordered. Laura was also referred to the Canberra Hearing Centre to have hearing tests.

None of the tests gave any idea of what was going wrong with Laura. Everything came back with no abnormalities found. No luck with the hearing tests either. The staff there could not tell if Laura was deaf, or simply not responding. Personally, we never felt that she was deaf. She still had a fair number of words, and those words she could say clearly.

The pediatrician also made an appointment for us to see a pediatric neurologist, who was coming down from Sydney to Canberra. The neurologist was to review the tests, and hopefully shed some light on the situation. We arrived to meet the neurologist at the time specified by her receptionist only to be told that we had missed our appointment. We knew that we did not have the wrong time, as we had had to schedule the appointment around Mark's preschool time. The neurologist, however, refused to see us and told us that we would either have to wait for 6 weeks for another appointment or go to Sydney.

Luckily, a different neurologist came to Canberra the following week. He made arrangements for Laura to be admitted into the Prince of Wales Children's Hospital in Sydney in March 1993. Laura was to undergo a battery of tests—more blood tests, rectal and skin biopsies, lumbar puncture, nerve conduction tests, and a brainstem evoked response hearing test. The latter would tell us for certain how well she could hear. We also met with a psychologist at the hospital. After observing Laura for a morning, she thought that Laura did not appear to be autistic, although she definitely had problems. We met the neurologist at that time too. He informed us that there was only about a 50% chance of finding the cause of Laura's regression. He also warned us that Laura might lose her gross motor skills.

Sure enough, the results of Laura's tests did not find any reason for her regression. It was devastating to still not know what was going on. Still more upsetting was the doctors' apparent lack of interest. No further help was offered, other than referral to an Early Intervention Center, and no further appointments were made. We were left with a child who wanted as little as possible to do with us.

Soon after all of these tests had been performed, in March 1993, Laura's condition seemed to stabilize somewhat. She began to tantrum less, and perhaps became more accepting of her disabilities. By this time, she was left with only limited speech and understanding; she preferred to stay on her own. She was preoccupied with repetitive rather than imaginative or purposeful activity.

In April 1993, a family friend saw a television report about a little boy with Landau–Kleffner syndrome (LKS), a rare form of epilepsy in which a child with previously normal development loses language skills and, to a greater or lesser degree, develops autistic symptoms. After the TV station supplied a free copy of the report to us, we felt that the symptoms appeared too similar to Laura's to dismiss. After doing some investigating of our own, we again approached the pediatric neurologist. We discovered that Laura had only had an ordinary EEG at the local hospital, not an extended sleep and awake EEG (commonly used to screen for LKS) and not with amitriptyline, a drug that is supposed to elicit abnormalities typical of LKS. The pediatric neurologist must have had several phone calls from other parents who had seen the report, because he was not impressed when we suggested it as a possibility for Laura. Laura had already had an EEG and there was nothing on it of any importance, he argued. Not an extended sleep and awake EEG with amitriptyline, we responded. An hour later he phoned back, apologized, and invited us to bring Laura back to Sydney for an extended sleep and awake EEG.

It was important to us to be certain Laura did not have LKS because we had heard that there was some possibility of a cure, especially if discovered early. Corticosteroids were being used successfully in a number of cases, and a U.S. doctor was having considerable success with surgery.

Unfortunately, the EEG did not show any evidence of LKS; we were still no wiser. After this extended EEG, the pediatric neurologist did not offer any explanation of what might be wrong with Laura, or any medical treatment. He also declined an offer to view a 7-minute video of Laura before and after her regression, which had been specially prepared for him.

In June 1993, Laura was to start attending a playgroup at an Early Intervention Centre. She was also offered one occupational therapy session, and one speech therapy session a fortnight. The first playgroup session was a disaster. Laura threw a huge tantrum. Within 5 minutes, we were with the doctor at the center. In one respect, the tantrum was a good thing. This doctor was quite helpful, and referred Laura to a psychologist to diagnose autism, or something else.

Laura attended the playgroup and speech and occupational therapy sessions for only one term, as they only catered to children aged 3 years and younger. Although it was only a short stay, it gave school counselors the opportunity to observe Laura and suggest the next best placement for her. We were keen to move her on from the Early Intervention Centre too, as such limited sessions gave little hope for achieving much.

In August 1993, we had our first appointment with the psychologist. She was going to observe Laura in several surroundings to get a clearer picture of her problems. We had also our video footage showing Laura before, during, and after regression. This video footage has proved invaluable to us.

In September, the psychologist offered a diagnosis. Laura presented as autistic but, for a number of reasons, was diagnosed with

"Other Childhood Disintegrative Disorder" as described in ICD-10—the 10th edition of the *International Classification of Diseases,* published by the World Health Organization.[1] In explaining her diagnosis to us, the psychologist told us that there were factors suggesting that Laura's diagnosis should not be simply "autism." These were her "flashes of normalcy" when she interacted with us, and the impression that she was in some way aware of her problems (which was not characteristic of autism), as well as the late onset of the disorder after a period of normal development.

Although we had been bracing ourselves for an autistic disorder, this was still a terrible blow. It seemed so final, and life seemed to hold little or no hope. It seemed as if we had lost a child, as in a sense we have.

Laura does seem to us to fit the diagnostic guidelines for CDD, as outlined in ICD-10. In particular, her early development was completely normal. Only after the age of 2 years did she lose previously learned skills, and acquired deficits and abnormalities in social interaction, communication, and behavior. The description of CDD in ICD-10 gives an even bleaker prognosis than that for autism. It is stated that after initial regression, although there may be some limited improvement, this will not continue and the child will be left with profound disability.

Despite the initial shock of the diagnosis, we did not lose hope that Laura might be able to make a significant improvement. It was clear that although its recent establishment as a separate diagnostic entity might be based on sound observations, CDD was a poorly understood condition, and in some ways little more than a label to describe children who had undergone an autistic regression after normal early development.

Later, by chance we were able to make contact with the parents of another CDD child in Australia—Jenny and Fred Fairthorne of Perth—and from that fortuitous contact, we learned of others in the "CDD network." Jenny has been, and continues to be, a great help to us. She has sent us papers about CDD, referred us to Jenny Bolland, the excellent "educator of autistic children" who has worked with her son David, given us information that has been instrumental in obtaining treatment and tests, and compared notes with us about CDD.

Having read more about CDD, we wrote to international experts on CDD and other developmental disorders, such as Dr. Hiroshi Kurita of the University of Tokyo, Professor Fred Volkmar of Yale University Medical School, Professor Isabelle Rapin of Albert Einstein College in New York, Dr. Rosenbloom in Liverpool, and Dr. Thierry Deonna in Lausanne. The replies confirmed that a child with CDD, once regression has taken place, is in many ways indistinguishable from a child with autism, and suggested that we seek to have Laura educated in the same way as an autistic child. Unfortunately, the international experts could not suggest anything more regarding treatment, nor could they give us much more insight into a possible cause for Laura's regression.

Meanwhile, we had gradually developed a suspicion that Laura's regression might have been triggered by the vaccination she had received in early October 1992 against *Haemophilus influenzae* type B (ProHIBiT vaccine). Before Laura had had the vaccination, on her grandparents' advice, we had asked the administering doctor whether it was safe to proceed, as Laura had severe eczema. However, when Laura's regression began, we did not immediately make any connection, because no acute event had followed the vaccination.

The LKS information pack, which we received in April 1993, included a leaflet from the National Vaccine Information Center in the United States. The leaflet described severe adverse reactions to vaccines. This made Laura's grandparents wary that Laura's regression may have been related to the vaccination, but they did not consider the possibility seriously at the time. Their suspicions were somewhat further aroused after professionals failed to offer any further tests or medical treatment after Laura's extended EEG in Sydney in May 1993. These suspicions strengthened about September 1993 after reviewing video records. From recollections of family members, we were able to establish that within 2 weeks of the vaccination she was failing to respond to family members and running around aimlessly.

Our suspicions were strengthened when we learned of serum sickness reactions and vasculitis associated with vaccinations. We began to learn of significant numbers of children experiencing regression similar to Laura's after vaccination, particularly through families in the United Kingdom. A number of vaccination information groups reported families with children regressing in a similar way to Laura, but none could offer any causal mechanism.

At this time, we managed to obtain Laura's medical records, and compared them with the home videos. We found that Laura had had eczema within a few days after at least two of her four triple antigen in-jections (at 2 and 18 months). She also acquired oral thrush after the first triple antigen at 2 months, and developed a lump behind one ear after the second at 4 months. These findings appeared to show a history of reactions to vaccines.

In September 1993, Laura underwent a brain magnetic resonance imaging (MRI). Like a CAT scan, MRI can detect structural abnormali-ties in the brain, and MRI can often distinguish a greater level of detail. However, Laura's MRI showed no abnormalities.

Because we had heard of cases where children with LKS did not show the signs of LKS on their EEGs until some time after onset of the disorder, we asked for a second extended awake and sleep EEG. This was performed in November 1993. The EEG showed minor irregulari-ties ("occasional sharp wave forms in mild excess") in the frontal re-gions, but no definite epileptic activity and no signs suggestive of LKS, or the similar "acquired epileptic frontal syndrome" (also known as the "syndrome of epileptic status in slow-wave sleep" (ESSS) or Tassinari syndrome).

In January 1994, frustrated with our lack of progress with main-stream medicine, we sought the advice of an osteopath who had been recommended to us. He claimed that Laura was not autistic, and that he might be able to help her by practicing regular osteopathic manipula-tion on her, namely, putting pressure on various points around her head. He explained that the aim of this was to correct a presumed im-balance in the brain. Although we were not certain about the validity of this treatment, we perceived that we and Laura had nothing to lose. We decided to proceed.

Laura had weekly "manipulation" sessions from January through April 1994. In the first week or two, we thought we saw some improve-ment, although it was difficult to be sure, particularly given that at the same time we had decided to be firmer in controlling Laura's behavior (we had come to the conclusion that, with her increasingly frequent tantrum-ing, we had become too accommodating). After this, however, we ob-served no further improvement. At one stage, the osteopath gave Laura a single dose of thuja, a homeopathic medicine often used as an "antidote" to problems caused by vaccination. This also had no apparent effect.

We had read that neurological problems are sometimes caused by cerebrovascular disorders (affecting the blood vessels in the brain) such as systemic lupus erythematosus (SLE). Among these disorders is isolated cerebral angiitis of the central nervous system, which cannot always be detected by the tests that Laura had undergone. Cerebrovascular disorders may be evaluated by means of angiography, which involves injecting contrast material (dye) into the bloodstream and tracking its progress through the brain, or by ultrasound ("transcranial Doppler ultrasound" in this case).

We were told, however, that angiography is an unpleasant procedure, and associated with risks. Ultrasound is noninvasive, but can detect only abnormalities in the major arteries of the brain, rather than the smaller ones that would be affected in a case of isolated cerebral angiitis. In view of the risks with angiography, we asked our pediatric neurologist for the ultrasound. Laura had the ultrasound in February 1994, and while in the hospital for this she also had some blood tests for cerebrovascular disorders. Both the ultrasound and the blood tests showed normal results.

In the meantime, regarding her education, Laura had started her three sessions a week at the local Autistic Unit in Canberra in September 1993. Her first term went quite well. She settled in well, although it took her quite some time to become accustomed to the routine. Laura still had some speech, although it was losing its purpose. She could also still sing a few songs, but she could not follow any instructions.

The Autistic Unit had eight places for children aged 3, 4, and 5 years. It was designed as a preschool, based on the TEACCH (Treatment and Education of Autistic and related Communication handicapped CHildren) program, as developed by Eric Schopler. It has a free play area, worktables, tables for structured play, and outside play areas. Four children attend at a time, with one teacher and one assistant. Children who have little or no speech are encouraged to communicate using "compic," simple drawings, or by photos. We could not say that Laura really achieved anything in that first term. Perhaps this was because she attended on Monday, Tuesday, and Wednesday, and the four subsequent days she spent basically forgetting everything she just learned! She was not unhappy there. The teacher managed to guide Laura through problems, and started to make attempts at toilet training. Unfortunately, Laura ignored these attempts and had many "accidents."

Major problems arose over the long, Christmas holiday, from December 1993 to January 1994. In Australia Christmas is in the summer, and children have a 6-week break. Many children with autistic spectrum disorders simply cannot cope with this change in routine. Things started to go downhill again, first evidenced when Laura started to refuse to wear one of her nighties. Naively we thought that this really did not matter; Laura had plenty of other clothes that she could wear. Gradually, however, Laura started to tantrum over other clothes too. There appeared to be no logical reason as to why she was behaving in this way but, if there is one thing that living with a child who presents as autistic has taught us, there is often no apparent reason for anything that child does.

In late January/early February school began again. This time Laura did not take kindly to going. There were many difficulties in separating from her mother, and many tantrums. Life was generally becoming very difficult again. Gradually Laura was objecting to more and more clothes; this behavior became worse and worse. We consulted the psychologist who had diagnosed Laura. She advised us to have a few sessions with a friend of hers, whose opinion she greatly valued, at a cost of $40 per session. We were becoming desperate. Despite concerns as to the value of these sessions, we proceeded. In three sessions, we were advised that we could either teach Laura gradually to accept the clothes that for some inexplicable reason were so offensive to her, or force her to wear what we chose—two quite obvious ideas to anyone. At the final session, Laura suddenly decided to take all of her clothes off again. We looked at each other, then at the two psychologists. We honestly thought that they would do something, show us what to do, or how far to push Laura, but they both sat in silence. That was the end of the sessions with those psychologists.

In early 1994, we were beginning to consider the possibility of arranging for Laura to undergo some form of intensive early intervention program. We had learned about these programs when relatives in the United Kingdom sent us a magazine report about the Higashi school— a school in Japan that has claimed remarkable success in treating autistic children with intensive behavior modification techniques. The school had a campus in Boston. We also learned through two different sources about the intensive programs being conducted under the auspices of O. Ivar Lovaas, a U.S. psychologist who had spent 25 years working on educational methods for autistic children. By chance we received an article from *Autism Research Review International*,[2] reporting that in their latest paper Lovaas and his co-workers had claimed that over 40% of autistic children whom they had put through an intensive program had not only returned to normal functioning, but retained their gains.[3] Almost at the same time, we received a video from Jenny and Fred Fairthorne in Perth that included footage of therapy sessions based on Lovaas's methods being administered to their son, David.

To us, what Lovaas said made sense: The way to go was to provide one-to-one help at first, in short, quick bursts of effort, up to at least 40 hours per week, and to use repetition, while keeping the program as interesting and motivating as possible. We were keen to arrange therapy for Laura that had some of these features, if not a full-blown Lovaas program.

By the end of that term the weather was becoming very cool, and Laura was wearing fewer and fewer clothes. Easter came and went, but there was no improvement. By the beginning of the next term, we were taking Laura out dressed only in a coat and a nappy. The final straw was when the coat was refused, too. The next day, Laura refused to wear even a nappy. She still was not toilet trained, and with two other young children, Mark $5\frac{1}{2}$ at the time and Joanna just 2 (and at the stage of wanting to copy her elder siblings!), life seemed almost impossible.

That day we finally phoned the Australian Capital Territory Health Minister's office. It was around 5 PM, and we could see no end to the mess we were in. We were worn out and depressed. We could not take much more. The Minister's office said they would send a social worker the next morning. "We don't want a social worker, we want help now," we said. "The social worker will be able to tell you what services are available," was the reply.

The social worker came the next morning. She was very sorry, but there were no services available. We were stunned. That statement destroyed any hope we had of improving our situation. We phoned the Minister's office again that day, and received a cursory response. The Minister was apparently involved in a scandal and was fighting for his political career. We were not sympathetic. Until he resigned he was still responsible for the lack of services.

Meanwhile, our other two children were terrified. While Laura was tantruming, Mark would hide under his bed. Joanna, who was not quite 2 at the time, was also frightened of Laura. We felt there was a real danger that, in her tantruming, Laura might hurt Joanna or Mark. Under these circumstances, we felt that we could not go on. That night (April 13, 1994), as there was nowhere else we could take her, we admitted Laura to the hospital. At the time she had a rash. Although she had been vaccinated for rubella $2\frac{1}{2}$ years earlier, her doctors were cautious about this possibility. Laura was, therefore, placed in isolation at the hospital.

It was unfortunate that we received the information requested from the Lovaas clinic detailing how to run an intensive early intervention program too late to be able to arrange for a program before Laura was admitted to the hospital. We received a first package of basic material in late March, just as Laura was going into crisis, and then a second package containing the Lovaas manual,[4] and a short videotape, after Laura's admission. If only we had known about the Lovaas program earlier, and received this material earlier, maybe Laura would have made greater gains sooner, and not had to leave home. Laura stayed in the hospital for 3 months. During this time she did not receive any treatment of any use until the third month. Being in an isolation ward, she was unable to leave her room for most of her stay. Although the nursing staff was very competent and caring, and we and Laura's grandparents visited for a number of hours each day, this period was undoubtedly another major step backward for her.

After Laura's admission, the president of the ACT Autism Association became involved. Having been through her own problems a few years earlier, she was able to give us useful advice. Our main concern was that we would lose our daughter. We had put her in the hospital, but did not know how long she would be there, or if she was going to be offered any treatment. We did not know what Welfare might do, or how they would view the situation.

The first appointment we had was with the Community Advocate. As far as they were concerned, Laura was their client, and their job was to ensure that Laura's needs were met. The second appointment we made was with Legal Aid. We were concerned that the hospital would make us take her home without giving her any treatment. Thus, we would be back to square one. Legal Aid confirmed that the hospital could not do anything like that once Laura had been admitted.

After Laura had been in the hospital for 1 week, a case conference was held. We were present, along with Laura's grandfather, her pediatrician, the nurse in charge of Laura's ward, a hospital social worker, and several people who provided respite services. It was quickly decided that the respite service placements were not suitable. They would not be able to cope with the scale of the problem. The pediatrician did not say much during the conference. We did note, however, who stayed and who did not to see the video of Laura "in action." The pediatrician did not stay.

At this time, we found out about the Behavior Intervention Team (BIT), a small unit under the Bureau of Community Services whose function was to assist with management of behavior problems. Because the BIT team was not allowed to come into institutions, they were not able to help Laura while she was in the hospital. This was ironic. If we had been informed earlier about the BIT team, when Laura was still at home, we might have been able to head off Laura's problems with clothes, and we might not have needed to admit her to the hospital.

Despite our making repeated pleas to the local authorities, very little happened with respect to deciding Laura's future, for the next few weeks. We approached the *Canberra Times,* and they ran a large article on Laura on May 14, 1994. It certainly helped to get the ball rolling. The local politicians at last started to show an interest in the case.

Despairing the lack of action from the local authorities, we finally decided to ask Jenny Bolland, the "educator of autistic children," to fly from Perth to set up an intensive early intervention program for Laura, based on Professor Lovaas's methods. She arrived on June 14.

Jenny was brilliant, as well as immensely dedicated to improving Laura's situation. Laura, though, did not especially appreciate her efforts. She was not interested in doing work of any kind and certainly did not share our respect for O. Ivar Lovaas! However, within the lone week that Jenny was in Canberra, Laura made major strides complying with instructions, and also showed interest in some of the tasks that she was being directed to complete. Early "compliance" tasks included "look at me," "clap hands," "stand up," and "sit down," among others. The task of matching one object to another was also begun that first week.

Things finally began to look up when we had a meeting with the Australian Capital Territory Minister for Community Services, David Lamont, and the newly appointed Minister for Health, Terry Connolly. The Chief Minister had seen the article in the *Canberra Times* and had said to her Ministerial colleagues that something ought to be done for Laura. Mr. Lamont, who had the main responsibility, told us that his department had proposed to him a treatment plan for Laura, but he had rejected it, because it was a "Band-Aid" solution. He was determined that we should be offered a long-term solution.

After this, the Bureau of Community Services, through the BIT team, finally got involved in Laura's case, and agreed to carry on with the intensive program Jenny Bolland had started. There were still many things to organize, however. It was decided that Laura should go into a government house in an attempt to reintroduce clothes. Clothes had been dotted around the hospital ward, but Laura had shown no real interest in them. We needed to start from scratch.

In July 1994, Laura moved into the government house, with staff specifically rostered to look after her and administer the program. Almost immediately after the move, Laura was forced to wear clothes, starting with a one-piece outfit. After a few hours of tantruming, she gave in to wearing the new outfit on the very first day. After this, she began to wear other clothes. It appeared that the clothes problem had been solved, but in fact it lay dormant, as was to become evident later.

In a sense, we were fortunate that Laura's problems precipitated a crisis and media attention. The government became willing to commit considerable resources to treating Laura. Laura's crisis enabled us to have an intensive program, although it fell far short of what she truly needed. We began to appreciate that all children with CDD, autism, or similar problems should have access to intensive early intervention.

Laura stayed in the government house for 11 weeks, to become accustomed to wearing clothes again and to her intensive program. Although she still had tantrums, they were not of the magnitude of those she had had before going into the hospital. We agreed to take Laura back home, judging that we (particularly our other children) would now be able to cope. Laura came home on October 1, 1994. The BIT team continued Laura's intensive program in our home.

We found having a home-based program a two-edged sword. The program has been of immeasurable help to Laura, teaching her skills ranging from constructive play to preschool skills such as sitting cross-legged on the floor to listen to a story. The staff who worked directly with Laura displayed great enthusiasm and commitment. Nonetheless, it was a great burden having nonfamily members in the house for up to 30 hours per week, even though they were very sensitive to the need of the family for privacy. Unfortunately, this sensitivity was not always shared by the administrators responsible for supervising the program.

Although the government devoted many resources to the program, it did not select a supervisor with the necessary experience to actively review the program week by week, to keep it on track. (The need for such a supervisor is emphasized in the literature on intensive early intervention.) The professionals who supervised Laura's program were undoubtedly very able within their own field of expertise, but were clearly amiss with respect to Laura's very specific program when difficulties presented.

In the absence of a supervisor with the appropriate experience, the program lost direction soon after it began, and was not as effective as it could have been. In particular, little effort was made, at least until much later, to supplement the concentrated training of specific tasks ("Discrete Trial Training") with a broader educational program, or to generalize the specific tasks that Laura would need to learn for daily living.

To further explore possible causes of Laura's regression, and to find out if there were any other treatments that might help, in November 1994, we visited a GP with a special interest in nutrition. He arranged more blood tests for Laura, which showed that she had an extremely high level of IgE (an indicator of a very sensitive immune system) and an allergy to a number of common grasses. The blood sample taken from Laura also underwent a "cytotoxic food allergy test," which in itself is not regarded as reliable, but which the GP told us could point the way to options for elimination diets. This test showed possible allergies to pork and peanuts, and to a lesser extent a number of other foods, including wheat, potato, and egg white.

The GP concluded from these tests and from our description of Laura's history that Laura had a very sensitive immune system, which had been "overloaded" by vaccination. Over the next 4 months, the GP put Laura through a series of elimination diets, with nutritional supplements. The diets involved eliminating all artificial colorings and preservatives, foods containing amines (e.g., chocolate, cheese) and salicylates (e.g., corn-based products, broccoli), and foods to which Laura had tested as possibly allergic (e.g., pork and foods with wheat, egg, and potato). The salicylates, amines, and "suspect" foods were then reintroduced progressively over a period of time.

At the same time, Laura was given a wide range of dietary supplements, vitamins, and medication in various combinations over the 4 months: vitamins A, C, D, and E; evening primrose oil; zinc; *Lactobacillus acidophilus*/bifidobacteria; glutamine; methionione; calcium; and an antihistamine. Unfortunately, we observed no change in Laura. We were no wiser.

We had heard about testing that was being done by Dr. Rosemary Waring at the University of Birmingham in the United Kingdom on children with "allergy-induced autism." Dr. Waring and her associates had shown that many of these children have an abnormally low level of sulfates. The researchers hypothesized that the children lack an enzyme necessary to metabolize certain foodstuffs, thus leading to a buildup of toxic chemicals and affecting the functioning of the brain.[5] We arranged for urine and blood samples to be taken from Laura and sent to the University of Birmingham for analysis. Although her urine test suggested low sulfate levels, her blood test indicated that these levels were within the normal range. However, the tests also showed a high level of cysteine and a very high level of sulfite. Dr. Waring explained to us that a high level of cysteine (an "excitotoxin") can affect the functioning of a certain neurotransmitter, so that it is like having a light on inside the brain at all times. Further, the presence of a high level of sulfite, which is a toxic substance, could suggest low levels of molybdenum, or low levels of the enzyme sulfite oxidase, which are known to be associated with neurological problems. Dr. Waring noted that some of the other children with high levels of sulfite revealed some improvement after molybdenum was included in their diet, and suggested that we try this. This is currently on the list of treatments that we are considering.

We wonder if it is just coincidence that other children in the United Kingdom who appear to be sufferers of "allergy-induced autism" have also been found to have high levels of sulfite. Perhaps Laura's regression may have been caused by allergies, which are associated with a defective immune system. We cannot help but believe it significant that many other parents of children with "allergy-induced autism" also suspect that vaccination damaged their children's immune systems, causing regression.

We have begun trying to give Laura the dietary supplements "Super Nuthera" and dimethylglycine (DMG). Super Nuthera contains a number of vitamins and nutritional supplements, but the main ingredients are vitamin B_6 and magnesium. A large number of controlled studies have shown that vitamin B_6/magnesium improves the functioning of a significant proportion of persons with autism.[6,7] Both B_6/magnesium and DMG are rated highly as to their effectiveness in questionnaires completed by parents of autistic children compiled by the Autism Research Institute in San Diego, directed by Dr. Bernard Rimland.

Unfortunately, subsequent to trying to give Laura dietary supplements in February 1995, she has become very resistant to taking anything that looks like medicine. She will also not eat or drink anything that looks or tastes different from a very restricted range of foods and drinks. We have not managed to entice Laura to take enough of either supplement to determine whether there is any benefit.

After Laura's home-based program was completed in January 1996, we turned our attention back to seeing if we could find a medical cause and, hopefully, a medical treatment for Laura's disorder. We were particularly interested in the possibility of treatment with immunoglobulin or corticosteroids.

Immunoglobulin therapy has been pioneered by Dr. Sudhir Gupta, professor of neurology at the University of California at Irvine. He has now treated at least 25 persons with autism, with good results.[8] One notable success has been the case of a boy in the United States who was found to have abnormally high levels of antirubella antibodies, suggesting that his autistic regression was caused by an adverse reaction to an earlier vaccination against rubella. He has now resumed normal functioning, apparently as a result of the immunoglobulin therapy. Because of the indications of abnormalities in Laura's immune system, we came to consider immunoglobulin therapy as an option for treatment for Laura.

Corticosteroid treatment has been administered by a number of neurologists to children thought to have LKS or the related acquired epileptic frontal syndrome. Recently, Dr. Gerry Stefanatos, a neurologist at Jefferson Medical College in Philadelphia, has treated successfully a number of children who failed to show signs of these disorders on regular testing (extended awake and sleep EEG), but who did show abnormalities suggestive of LKS on further specialized testing.[9] Laura had exhibited minor irregularities on EEG testing, but not signs specifically suggestive of either LKS or acquired epileptic frontal syndrome. Given the delays and difficulty involved in arranging the specialized testing employed by Dr. Stefanatos, we were considering requesting a trial course of corticosteroids in any case. However, we have now received a reply from Dr. Stefanatos advising us that Laura does not appear to have LKS and that the additional tests are not required.

Before requesting our pediatrician to begin either of these treatments, we felt it might be useful to have additional tests performed. We arranged for a third extended sleep and awake EEG; tests for levels of the various types of immunoglobulin in the blood; tests for antibodies to the diseases against which Laura had been vaccinated; and a skin patch test for sensitivity to thimerosal, a preservative commonly used in the HIB and "triple antigen" vaccines.

The EEG this time showed no abnormalities. We took this to indicate that if Laura's disorder was associated with abnormal epileptic discharges, either those discharges had by now ceased, or they had been taking place at a very deep level in the brain—too deep to detect now, at least without using highly invasive techniques.

Immunoglobulin testing in March 1996 showed that Laura still had a very high level of IgE. As mentioned earlier, this suggests that Laura has a general tendency toward allergies, and is to be expected in children who have had eczema within the previous 2 years. However, the result was perhaps a little surprising, considering that Laura had been without eczema for over 2 years. Levels of other immunoglobulins—IgA, IgM, IgG, and IgG subclasses—were normal or near normal.

Tests for antibodies to the diseases against which Laura had been vaccinated showed that Laura had not developed immunity to any of these diseases from the vaccine. She had no antibodies to whooping cough or mumps and, though she tested with antibodies to rubella, we believe this was a result of having contracted the disease in early 1994, long after having been vaccinated against rubella. Levels of antibodies to measles also suggested that she had in fact contracted the disease. Antibodies to hemophilus influenzae type B (HIB), tetanus, and polio were insufficient to confer immunity.

Dr. Reed Warren of Utah State University and his co-workers have shown that autism is associated with altered resistance to infection, and that in some cases a child with autism will fail to respond to immunization.[10,11] There have also been reports of children who appear to have developed autism as a result of an excessive reaction to an immunization.[12]

It seems to us that we could interpret these antibody results in three ways. First, they could simply be coincidental and unrelated to

Laura's regression. Second, we could suppose that Laura did not form antibodies because she had an inborn inability to respond normally to immune system challenges, associated with a latent autistic spectrum disorder. Finally, however, we could hypothesize that Laura had immune system abnormalities that put her at risk if vaccinated, and that on HIB vaccination triggered her autistic regression.

Laura also had a skin patch test to determine whether she was hypersensitive to thimerosal, a mercury-based substance used as a preservative in a number of vaccines, including ProHIBiT and diphtheria–pertussis–tetanus (DPT) vaccines. We requested this test as review of Laura's medical records suggested that she might have had adverse reactions after at least two of her four DPT vaccinations. We wondered if Laura might have become sensitized to thimerosal, to the extent that finally the ProHIBiT vaccination precipitated her regression. The test, however, was negative. Nonetheless, we feel it remains to be shown that Laura could not have had a hypersensitivity or toxic reaction to a component of the ProHIBiT vaccine—perhaps the diphtheria toxoid, which is also a component of the DPT vaccine.

After these tests, we visited our pediatrician to discuss possible treatment with either immunoglobulin or corticosteroids. We were neutral about which would be better to try first. The pediatrician explained that, in view of the associated risks and, in the case of immunoglobulin, the shortage of medication, he would have to go through special procedures to initiate treatment. He noted that the risks were greater with corticosteroids, and that it might therefore be preferable to explore the possibility of immunoglobulin treatment first. He then obtained agreement from our local hospital to make gammaglobulin available, and had us sign a disclaimer. In May 1996, Laura started on a trial course of eight gammaglobulin infusions, to be administered once every 3 weeks.

At the time of this writing, Laura has had seven of the eight gammaglobulin infusions. The treatment has largely coincided with a relatively "good" period for Laura. She has been somewhat more responsive to other people, and more interested in cognitive activities such as puzzles, matching letters, and using photographs to communicate. However, the improvement is not dramatic, and may well have begun just before the gammaglobulin therapy was initiated. There has also been a possible negative effect. Laura's toilet training has taken a step backward. We intend to monitor Laura's progress over the full trial period, and consult with our pediatrician regarding continuing treatment after that.

While we have been pursuing the immunoglobulin therapy, we have become aware of other suggestions for treatment. The Defeat Autism Now! manual,[13] produced as a result of a major conference in the United States, includes among its options a trial of multiple nutrients with an emphasis on calcium and selenium, as well as vitamin B_6, magnesium, and zinc. This may be worth trying. Selenium has also been suggested to us by another professional.

The same professional also suggested trying a treatment of coenzyme Q and/or NOOTROPIL tablets. As yet we do not know much about these treatments. We understand that coenzyme Q has been used with children with neurological disorders, and is available in tablet form. NOOTROPIL tablets are designed to aid blood circulation in the brain. The professional also mentioned tests that we could put Laura through before trying the above treatments. The Defeat Autism Now! manual refers to a wide range of diagnostic tests, including a complete immunological investigation and testing for levels of various minerals. We believe that some of these may also be worth considering in the future.

Finally, a homeopath has been recommended to us who claims considerable success in treating children with autistic symptoms, including with vaccine damage. We have gone through an initial assessment with this homeopath, and he has proposed some treatment. At the time of writing, we are not sure about the nature and basis of this treatment, and have therefore not proceeded further.

Although Laura's intensive home-based program has ended, and she now attends full time at a special school for children with many kinds of disabilities, we have tried to make sure that Laura continues to obtain some educational intervention at home. We have been fortunate in that one of the therapists who worked with Laura in her intensive program (very effectively) has continued working with her during school holidays, under a government "individual support package," and also throughout the year as a home-based respite care worker. We also do as much as we can to try to get Laura to use her time constructively and develop her skills. This is often difficult, as we are usually faced with demands for attention from our two other children, while Laura is mostly busy avoiding attention.

What Laura Is Like Now

Laura's progress has continued to be mixed. Since she returned home in October 1994, she has responded slowly but steadily to her home-based program, and her sessions at the autistic preschool. Previously it was almost impossible to get her to do anything, now she will often follow simple instructions to sit down, stand up, and pick up objects (although her level of compliance varies). She will play with puzzles, blocks, and a limited range of other toys. She will also sometimes join in or initiate simple play with others, and give family members cuddles and "kisses." She can also communicate to a very limited degree, with prompting, by nodding or shaking her head to say "yes" or "no." At times she will take a photograph of something she wants and give it to an adult; and, more recently, she has begun taking an adult by the hand to the object or activity she desires.

Since coming home, Laura has had more crises involving clothes. In January 1995, she began to again refuse to wear tops. To get her to wear anything, we had to hold her for hours while she tantrumed wildly. We were able to defuse this crisis when, after a number of weeks, we succeeded in getting her to wear some cream-colored tops Sue had sewn. In mid-1995, we had a similar crisis, with further eruptions in late 1995 and January 1996, with pants, shorts, and shoes, respectively. Tantrums now often involve Laura biting and scratching herself or others, or Laura banging her head on the floor.

Apart from the problems with clothes, Laura also creates major headaches in public. She persistently runs off when Sue is picking up our eldest son from school, and taking her shopping or elsewhere can quickly result in tantrums.

At the onset of Laura's regression, she could speak well for her age (2 years 3 months). Even after her regression, she retained speech and singing for some months. However, over time her speech has disappeared, and now only very rarely will she even say a recognizable word (mostly "no"). Although she will occasionally participate in play, either by herself or with others, the time spent this way is a very small portion of her total waking hours; the rest is dominated by self-stimulatory activity. Inside, she likes to find an object to carry with her. Outside, she likes to pick up sand or dirt to feel and carry, and, if not stopped, to eat.

Much of the time Laura is happy. She is capable of enjoying things such as eating, drinking, swimming, jumping on the trampoline, swinging, watching videos, and joining in rough-and-tumble play. However, compared with a normal child, the quality of her life is very poor, and her problems affect the entire family and extended family. Because of this, we want to confirm the cause of her regression; to try treatments, whether medical, behavioral, or educational, that may improve her prospects; and to prevent the same from happening to other children.

Lessons from Laura

In the preceding pages, we have tried to set out our experiences with Laura, from her birth to the present. We would also like to add our thoughts on the cause of Laura's regression; on the various treatments that we have tried or are contemplating; and on how parents can get help for their children with CDD, be it with treatment, tests, or funding for behavioral/educational programs.

Apart from our own experience, there are a number of reasons why we believe that vaccination may be one cause underlying autistic spectrum disorders, including CDD. First, although there has been little systematic work in this area, there are a few studies suggesting that there may be a link. These include work published in the peer-reviewed professional literature,[14] as well as a recent preliminary study performed under the auspices of the Developmental Delay Registry, a group formed by parents to promote research on, and identify treatments for, development delay.[15] In addition, reports in the literature show that a significant number of parents of autistic children consider vaccination to be associated with autism in their children.[16]

In an issue of the *Autism Research Review International,* the newsletter of the Autism Research Institute in San Diego, autism researcher and Institute Director Dr. Bernard Rimland suggests that there is increasing evidence that many autistic children become autistic soon after receiving a vaccination.[17] He calls for further research on the possible connection between vaccination and autistic spectrum disorders. This is precisely what we believe is needed. Parents of children with autistic spectrum disorders need to know whether to have their children vaccinated further, and other parents need to be able to make a fully informed decision on whether to vaccinate their children. We believe that there is a need for carefully structured large-scale studies on the possible connection between vaccination and autistic spectrum disorders.

Treatment

The only treatment that was clearly beneficial for Laura was the intensive early intervention program. Although Laura's program has not enabled her to return to normal functioning, as it has for many children treated by the Lovaas clinic, it has helped to improve her functioning in a range of areas, and has provided her with a solid basis on which to build in the future. This suggests to us that other children with CDD would also benefit greatly from such programs, even though they might be based on programs designed to treat autistic or other developmentally disabled children. This is despite the opinion expressed in some of the literature on CDD, that the deficits of these children are so severe that they show little response to treatment. Perhaps in the past investigators only looked at the more severe cases of CDD, as less severely affected children escaped the diagnosis.

Considerable success has been achieved with intensive early intervention for children with autism. Caring for autistic persons in later life is very costly if a substantial functional improvement has not been realized earlier in life.[18] We suggest that intensive early intervention is worth the effort for children with autism, and also for children with CDD.

Intensive early intervention programs, however, are few and far between in Australia. We know of only three cities on the continent with these programs. Worse, professionals do not, as a matter of course, mention these programs as a possible treatment to parents of CDD or autistic children. We believe that parents need to be informed about these programs.

There seems to be a widespread reluctance among professionals to diagnose an autistic spectrum disorder before the age of 3 years. It has been shown in a number of recent studies, however, that with careful monitoring, the emergence of autistic symptoms can be detected much earlier—at 18 months of age, or younger.[19]

Just as it can be difficult to obtain an early diagnosis, it can be hard to obtain a quick one. Our experience demonstrated that even if a child's family spots a problem immediately, it can take months or years to convince professionals. It is widely recognized that behavioral intervention needs to be commenced as early as possible. We believe that greater awareness of the disorder is needed, and that all children should be monitored for the emergence of autistic symptoms. Once such symptoms become evident, parents should be offered intensive early intervention programs for their children.

Lovaas stresses the importance of conducting early intervention programs in the child's natural environment (e.g., at home). We felt that we had to attempt the home-based program, for Laura's sake. However, it was very stressful for our other children and ourselves. It interrupted our other family activities, and deprived us of much needed privacy. We felt particularly so, because those responsible for supervising our program did not account for the other needs of the family. We suggest that these be taken into account in designing such programs.

We would like to stress the importance of having a good program supervisor in intensive early intervention programs. From our experience, it does not seem to be important for a supervisor to have formal qualifications, although clearly it may help to have a background in special education or psychology. It seems to us that the key qualities required for a good supervisor are experience with intensive early intervention programs; understanding of, and belief in, such programs; and the energy and enthusiasm to keep reviewing the program week by week to ensure that it remains fresh and directed to the needs of the child.

If no individual is available with these qualities, we suggest that families consider the possibility of supervising programs themselves. We do not, however, wish to underestimate the very great burden this would create for the family, in addition to their responsibilities for other children, work, and so on. Partly because of these considerations, we never attempted to run Laura's program by ourselves. In hindsight, perhaps we should have taken it over when it started to lose some of its direction. We suggest it may be preferable to run a program oneself, even if in a limited manner, rather than depend on someone who does not understand intensive programs or does not have the ability to work on keeping the program up to the mark week after week.

Apart from behavioral intervention, we have tried, looked into, or at least thought of medical and dietary intervention; "alternative" medical treatment; and other therapies such as auditory training and structured listening. It seems to us that because Laura and other CDD children re-gressed after a period of normal development, there should be a better chance that some form of treatment can make a difference than if they had been autistic from birth. Something happened to damage Laura's brain, and just maybe we can find some way of reversing the damage.

Under "medical intervention" falls the trial of gammaglobulin therapy that Laura is undertaking at the time of writing. We believed this was worth trying because Laura had some immunological abnor-malities, and because the therapy apparently has been effective in treat-ing a number of children with autism, including one whose immunological test results were suggestive of vaccine damage. There is some risk associated with the therapy, but we believed the potential benefit outweighed this risk. We have also been influenced by the in-creasing interest in the association of immunological abnormalities with autistic disorders.[20–24]

Another treatment that we have been considering is corticosteroid therapy—in case Laura has LKS or acquired epileptic frontal syndrome. We have now been advised that it is unlikely Laura has LKS, and we are, therefore, unlikely to try this treatment. However, this line of in-quiry is one that other parents might want to pursue. An additional point is that corticosteroids act to ease inflammation and suppress the immune system. If the mechanism underlying CDD in a particular child were an autoimmune disorder or encephalitis (inflammation of the brain), then this could be an additional rationale for employing corti-costeroids. Corticosteroids are sometimes used for treating neurological disorders with autoimmune characteristics, and encephalitis. Cortico-steroid treatment, however, carries considerable risks and side effects, and we suggest it would be advisable to learn about these before re-questing such treatment.

To treat autistic spectrum disorders, many persons have suggested dietary supplements. As mentioned earlier, we have tried elimination diets, and a range of supplements including vitamins, zinc, glutamine, and an antihistamine. We have yet to give a proper trial to vitamin B_6–magnesium supplementation or to DMG. A number of other addi-tives have been suggested as being useful, including selenium and vit-amin B_{15}. In addition, Laura's abnormally high level of sulfite suggests a trial of molybdenum. We believe that all of these suggestions are worth taking seriously.

It has also been suggested to us to try coenzyme Q (sometimes used in children with neurological disorders) or NOOTROPIL tablets, which are believed to enhance blood circulation in the brain. We are looking into these suggestions.

We have also tried alternative medical treatments, in the form of osteopathic manipulation and homeopathic medicine. Despite some initial encouraging signs with osteopathy, neither treatment was of any help. We found that, although the practitioners involved were well meaning, their explanations of the treatments were relatively unconvincing. We are now skeptical of the merits of such "alternative" approaches. However, vaccination group researchers have recommended that we consult a good homeopath, suggesting that such practitioners have had some success in treating cases of vaccine damage. It has also been suggested that we consult a kinesiologist.

We are of the opinion that we should try anything that has a realistic chance of helping Laura. At some stage, though, we may decide that we cannot put her, or the rest of the family, through anything more. Alternative therapies, therefore, particularly homeopathy, remain on our list of treatments that we are looking into.

We have also heard that sensory integration and auditory training have produced good results in some children with autistic disorders. We have, however, seen surprisingly little information about what they actually involve. Perhaps sensory integration could help children like Laura, who are tactile defensive. Recent research by Dr. Sue Bettison, formerly of the Autism Research Institute in Sydney, suggests that "structured listening," involving listening through headphones to a variety of music with particular features, is equally effective as auditory training.[25] Although Laura does not appear to have hypersensitivity to sound (if anything, she fails to respond to sound stimuli), we would consider auditory training and structured listening among future treatment options.

How to Get Help

In attempting to access tests, treatment, support services, and funding for Laura, we have had some successes and some failures. We also learned a few lessons.

When talking to professionals, particularly medical professionals, about nonstandard tests and treatment, we found it helpful to do our "homework" first. We prepared by reading the medical literature, deciding in advance what we wanted to ask, and, when necessary, putting in writing what we wanted. At appointments, we obtained the best results by staying calm and paying due respect to the expertise of the professionals, but remaining firm about our desires when necessary.

In trying to access support services and funding, which is often not readily available, we found it makes a tremendous difference if one goes to the top, particularly at the political level, and also to the media. It is remarkable what change can occur when one is dealing with elected officials who have to explain to the public what services they are or are not providing to children with debilitating disorders and massive problems.

We have not explored legal means to obtain services. Court cases and "due process hearings" in the United States where families have obtained funding for Lovaas-style intensive programs appear to provide a basis for parents to force authorities to provide a truly "free and appropriate education" for their children. To what degree the initial successes these parents obtained in the United States might be repeated in other countries is unknown. However, the idea of using legal means to obtain intensive intervention is one that may well be worthwhile pursuing.

Finally, we believe it is very important for parents of CDD children to make contact with each other; to exchange information and experiences; and (as a group) to maintain contact with professionals with expertise on CDD. Professionals and parents should work together to improve understanding of this baffling disorder, and hopefully develop new treatments. We have found our contacts in the International CDD Network invaluable in obtaining information, and sometimes crucial in obtaining treatment. If more parents join the Network, the information that could be obtained simply by compiling the histories of each child might be of great help to professionals with an interest in CDD.

We believe it is important for CDD parents, as a group if not individually, to maintain contact with support groups for disorders closely related to CDD, particularly autism. Such groups include: the Allergy-induced Autism Support and Research Network (U.K. and USA), CAN (Cure Autism Now) International, and the Developmental Delay Registry (USA). Given that the number of cases of diagnosed CDD is small, and that CDD is so similar to late-onset autism, it is also prudent to remain familiar with autism research.

Given the current state of knowledge about CDD, we believe it imperative to gather more information and conduct further research on this disorder, in our "quest for a cure."

Endnotes

1. World Health Organization, *International Classification of Diseases*, 10th ed., Geneva, 1992: pp. 256–257.
2. Rimland, B., "Long-term follow-up: Early intervention effects lasting," in *Autism Research Review International*, Vol. 7, No. 1, 1993: pp. 1, 6.
3. McEachin, J. J., Smith, T., and Lovaas, O. I., "Long-term outcome for children with autism who received early intensive behavioral treatment," in *American Journal on Mental Retardation*, Vol. 97, No. 4, 1993: pp. 359–372.
4. Lovaas, O.I., Ackerman, A.B., Alexander, D., Firestone, P., Perkins, J., and Young, D., *Teaching Developmentally Disabled Children: The "Me" Book*, Pro-Ed, Austin, TX, 1981.
5. O'Reilly, B.A., and Waring, R., "Enzyme and sulfur oxidation deficiencies in autistic children with known food/chemical intolerances," in *Journal of Orthomolecular Medicine* Vol. 8, No. 4, December 1993: pp. 198–200.
6. Gillberg, C., and Coleman, M., *The Biology of the Autistic Syndromes*, 2nd ed., Mackeith Press, London, 1992.
7. Rimland, B., "Studies of high dosage vitamin B6 in autistic children and adults—1965–1994," The Autism Research Institute, San Diego, 1994.
8. Goldenberg, C., Information package on gammaglobulin therapy available from the Autism Research Institute, San Diego (referred to in *Autism Research Review International*, Vol. 9, No. 2, 1995: p. 7).
9. Stefanatos, G.A., Grover, W., and Geller, E., "Case study: Corticosteroid treatment of language regression in pervasive developmental disorder," in *Journal of the American Academy of Child and Adolescent Psychiatry*, Vol. 34, No. 8, August 1995: pp. 1107–1111.
10. Warren, R.P., Singh, V.K., Cole, P., Odell, J.D., Pingree, C.B., Warren, W.L., DeWitt, C.W., and McCullough, M., "Possible association of the extended MHC haplotype B44-SC30-DR4 with autism," in *Immunogenetics*, Vol. 36, 1992: pp. 203–207.
11. Daniels, W.W., Warren, R.P., Odell, J.D., Maciulis, A., Burger, R.A., Warren, W.L., and Torres, A.R., "Increased frequency of the extended or ancestral haplotype B44-SC30-DR4 in autism," in *Neuropsychobiology*, Vol. 32, No. 3, 1995: pp. 120–123.

12. Baker, S.M., and Pangborn, J., "Clinical Assessment Options for Children with Autism and Related Disorders" (the "Defeat Autism Now!" manual), Autism Research Institute, San Diego, 1996.
13. Baker and Pangborn.
14. Tsaltas, M.O., "A pilot study on allergic responses," in *Journal of Autism and Developmental Disorders*, Vol. 16, 1986: pp. 91–92.
15. Dorfman, K., Lemer, P., and Nadeler, J., "What puts a child at risk for developmental delays?—Results of the Developmental Delay Registry survey": available from the Developmental Delay Registry, 6701 Fairfax Road, Chevy Chase, MD 20815.
16. Laxer, G., Rey, M., and Ritvo, E.R., "Brief report: A comparison of potentially pathologic factors in European children with autism, Down's syndrome, and multiple physical handicaps," in *Journal of Autism and Developmental Disorders*, Vol. 18, No. 2, 1988: pp. 309–313.
17. Rimland, B., "Is there an autism epidemic?" in *Autism Research Review International*, Vol. 9, No. 3, 1995: p. 3.
18. Lovaas, O.I., "Behavioral treatment and normal educational and intellectual functioning in young autistic children," in *Journal of Consulting and Clinical Psychology*, Vol. 55, No. 1, 1987: pp: 3–9.
19. Baron-Cohen, S., Allen, J., and Gillberg, C., "Can autism be detected at 18 months? The needle, the haystack and the CHAT," in *British Journal of Psychiatry*, Vol. 161, 1992: pp. 839–843.
20. Stubbs, E.G., Crawford, M.L., Burder, D.R., and Vandenbark, A.A., "Depressed lymphocyte responsiveness in autistic children," in *Journal of Autism and Childhood Schizophrenia*, Vol. 7, 1977: pp. 49–55.
21. Warren, R.P., Margaretten, N.C., Pace, N.C., and Foster, A., "Immune abnormalities in patients with autism," in *Journal of Autism and Developmental Disorders*, Vol. 16, 1986: pp. 189–197.
22. Warren, R.P., Foster, A., and Margaretten, N.C., "Reduced natural killer cell activity in autism," in *Journal of American Child and Adolescent Psychiatry*, Vol. 26, 1987: pp. 333–335.
23. Warren, R.P., Oink, L.J., Burger, R.A., and others, "Deficiency of suppressor inducer (CD4 + CD45RA +) T cells in autism," in *Immunological Investigations*, Vol. 19, 1990: pp. 245–251.
24. Warren, R.P., Singh, V.K., Cole, P., Odell, J., Pingree, C.B. , Warren, W.L., and White, E., "Increased frequency of the null allele at the complement C4B locus in autism," in *Clinical and Experimental Immunology*, Vol. 83, 1991: pp. 438–440.
25. Bettison, S., "Abnormal responses to sound and the long-term effects of a new treatment program," in Building Bridges: Proceedings of the 1995 National Autism Conference (Australia), Autistic Children's Association of Queensland (Inc.), Brisbane, 1995: pp. 25–40.

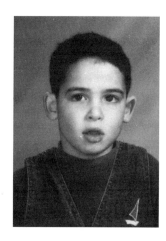

Seven

Looking for Answers
Chronicles of an Autistic Child

by Candice Goldstein

When I look at my 8-year-old son, Ben, profoundly retarded, still in diapers and unable to speak, I wonder. Were we lucky that at one time he seemed so bright? Or were we cursed? Unlike parents who are told at their child's birth that their infant son or daughter will "always have difficulties," we lived for years having high expectations for Ben. He was a bright, responsive infant. He seemed to progress normally.

I felt I might be pregnant with Ben a week or two after he was conceived. It was my first pregnancy and I was so excited. My husband, Abraham Steinberg, a urologist, and I were visiting Colorado from our home in Geneva, Illinois (40 miles from Chicago), for a long weekend that coincided with Abe's birthday and Valentine's Day. I went downhill and cross-country skiing and felt great. As soon as we returned, I called the doctor's office to schedule a pregnancy test. Anxious about waiting, I immediately began taking prenatal vitamins. The test confirmed what I already knew. At age 34, and after a year and a half of marriage, we were about to embark on a new adventure.

The first trimester did not go smoothly. Although I never suffered nausea and did not find it hard to continue working as an attorney in

Chicago, I had some bleeding, which seemed to be caused by infected cysts. I also needed a short course of antibiotics, and because of low progesterone levels, progesterone suppositories.

At about 12 weeks, I underwent a CVS sampling at Illinois Masonic Hospital. We received the results a few weeks later. None of the conditions the lab tested for, such as Down syndrome or other chromosomal abnormalities, were present. The last two trimesters proceeded uneventfully, although I avoided concentrated sweets because of elevated blood sugar.

My due date came and went. I was induced 10 days later—Saturday, October 28, 1989—and Ben was born. It was a wonderful feeling! Ben had a few physical abnormalities but the pediatrician at the hospital was not concerned about them and, reassured, I decided not to worry. His mouth twisted to the side when he cried, and he had trouble latching on to my breast when I tried to nurse him. My sister immediately dubbed him "Popeye" and "Buddy Hackett." Ben's ears not only protruded, but they seemed somewhat inelegant. A second pediatrician confirmed that they were missing a fold. Also, the indentation of skin above his buttocks was crooked, not straight. This, we were told, was a normal variant. Finally, when Ben was 3, a doctor examining him noted an indentation at the top of his chest, suggesting that his rib cage had never fully joined.

Although Ben still wasn't nursing well, we went home Monday morning. It took a week and a visit from a lactation consultant to finally establish nursing. At 8 days of age, Ben was ready for his *bris,* the Jewish ritual circumcision ceremony. I cried more than Ben. Pride over his bravery and stoicism consumed me.

By the end of his first month, Ben was looking at himself in a mirror we had put on his changing table. Not long after that, he was smiling at himself with his crooked little grin, and then at me, Abe, and anyone else. He cried less and less. He seemed more mature than other babies—more social eye contact, more smiles, and more in control. It was an easy decision to quit my full-time job and work part-time at home writing a legal periodical.

At the end of December, Ben contracted a cold, distinguished by an immutable cough and runny nose. The pediatrician observed that his eardrums were pink and prescribed an antibiotic. Ben hated it—he choked it down and sometimes vomited. Tylenol drops and the oral polio vaccine had the same effect. Taking medication by mouth continued to be a problem for the next year or so.

The remainder of the winter, Ben was a joy to care for. He was no problem in the car: He relaxed in the car seat, crossed his hands on his stomach, and away we would go. We received a Mylar balloon as a gift and attached it to his wrist while he laid on his back. He happily observed it float above him. However, he did not care for rattles and plastic teether toys. In fact, his videos show him using his hands very little. His first formal portrait taken at 3 months shows a baby smiling so hard his eyes curl. He recovered from all of the mishaps of babyhood with aplomb: sleeping in other babies' cribs when we went visiting, sliding out of the stroller, enjoying airplane travel, and other excitement.

By summer, he could stack plastic rings on a pole and play a toy organ. Getting him to wave, though, consumed great effort. He enjoyed "swimming" in a Styrofoam boat with a sling seat, and long walks in the stroller. He relished foods he could feed himself, Cheerios, chunks of fruit, French fries. At age 9 months, colic struck, and he began waking at night. After enduring a dreadful month, we forced Ben to "cry it out" at night and for naps. A week later peaceful sleep was reclaimed.

At his first birthday, Ben understood a few words and followed one-step directions. He consistently would bring us requested objects or toys. He especially liked to drop chain links into a bottle and stack rings. We were amused that in doing this he always used one or the other hand. The other was raised like a fencer's; never did Ben use both hands in a coordinated fashion. He could crawl well, but it would be several months before he could stand unassisted, and even longer before he could walk. He clung at first when we went somewhere new, but always warmed up after a few minutes. At 14 months, he could say bye-bye and give a stiff wave, but only with prompting. If we asked, "What does the doggy say?" he would say "ruf!" His singular bad habit was standing up in his highchair.

When he was about 18 months, I began taking Ben to a toddler fitness class. Ben seemed a little different than the other children his age. He was still drooling and was an unsteady walker, although he could climb and slide with the best of them. When the organized activities began, Ben seemed oblivious. The other toddlers could gather in a circle to sing "Itsy Bitsy Spider" and other finger plays, but Ben could not follow along or even clap to the music. However, unlike all of the children we came in contact with, he was always cheerful and never tantrumed when it was time to leave. In retrospect, Ben never said "da-da."

By his second birthday, Ben could point to pictures in his books in response to hearing an adult say "truck," "car," "baby," and "flower." He started to attend a toddler program at a Montessori school three mornings each week. He loved the toys, especially puzzles and peg-boards, the playground, and snacks. He had no trouble separating from me the first month, but began having difficulty the second. That soon passed. According to the other children's mothers, Ben was a favorite classmate. His interest in puzzles and shape games was admired by the adults, who perceived him as "smart." On the playground, he was sure-footed and never afraid to climb higher and higher. He didn't even cry when his swing flipped upside down and he dangled precariously for several minutes. Ben could point to each of his classmates in the class picture and say their names.

Ben, like several children in his class, contracted chickenpox that winter. Unlike them, he didn't seem particularly sick or even uncom-fortable. Until he started sneezing or coughing, I never could tell when Ben was about to come down with an illness. He was always smiling and cheerful.

The winter was distinguished by my terrific battle to keep gloves on Ben. I worried his hands would freeze on the playground and on the walks we took. I bought one pair of mittens after another, trying to find a pair from which Ben's hands would not slip. He seemed able to relax his hands so they would just fall off, or he would ease them off by rub-bing his mittened hands against his pants or coveralls. Tired from the battles, we took Ben to Florida. I noticed other young children on the beach filling buckets with sand and shells, but Ben preferred laying on his stomach on the warm sand. When his hands became sandy, he would not brush them off. Much sand was brought to his eyes and into his mouth. We took long walks along the beach, but he didn't seem to notice the birds, boats, or even me. If he ran ahead, he just went and went.

As our hotel room had a television with a VCR, I rented a video-tape of singers and dancers performing Mother Goose rhymes. Ben adored it. I also purchased a set of about 20 animal flashcards. Ben mas-tered these in a couple of sittings. He could take one card from the stack, name the animal, pick another, and so on, repeatedly.

When we returned, Ben developed a close friendship with another student at preschool. Among other things, they would chase each other around a wooden fort smiling and giggling. By year's end, Ben's teachers were impressed with his language acquisition. He was also finally able to assert himself. When others would try to take puzzles or toys from him he would protest, "No, my work." The teachers observed that Ben never seemed to be attracted to the practical living section of the classroom, where a sink, brooms, window spray, and other household items were kept. He spent most of his time with animal figures, books, and puzzles. He was able to work puzzles of 50 pieces or more, but always with one hand. The other was sometimes raised, reminiscent of his infancy. He seemed fascinated by television shows like *Sesame Street* and *Barney.* While they played, he would excitedly run back and forth in front of the television, sometimes even running in place.

By spring, Ben still had not mastered many of the tasks that were assigned to the children in his class. He could not put on his coat, hat, or shoes, or pour his juice. He would sit in his little chair for the snack, but spills were common. He loved the weekly music activity and offered his suggestions for songs, but would never sing with the group. Despite knowing the words to many rhymes and songs, he would only speak them and would stop as soon as someone joined in. During "Old McDonald's Farm," he raced around gathering small farm animal figures and would suggest the next animal to be named by placing it on the piano saying, "How about the horse?" or "How about the pig?" According to the teachers, when other children needed to leave to use the toilet, Ben would push his way into the bathroom with them, and stay until they finished. They thought Ben was starting to get interested in toilet training, but he was so passive and nonverbal regarding self-care that I found this difficult to believe. The pediatrician suggested I bribe Ben with a promise of a toy after a week of dry diapers, but I knew Ben could not understand the concept of a week's time or even dry diapers.

I missed the routine of school over the summer. Although Ben was very content to watch television or do puzzles, he did not play with other children. When we invited another child over, the other child's presence was not enough to keep Ben in the same room, or on the swing set. It seemed I had to keep chasing him back. Going on a hike, swimming, or going to the zoo seemed better. Although his friends were starting to ride tricycles, Ben could not master it. Like the other boys his age,

Ben liked to watch the cartoon, "Thomas the Tank Engine," and could push toy trains around a wooden track, but he was not creating scenarios like his friends. I noticed it was still easier to serve Ben his meals in a highchair, a restriction other children would not allow. Further, I had to cut Ben's sandwiches and pizza into small pieces; he could not manage a large piece.

One exciting moment came after Ben awoke from a nap and asked, "Where's Betty [the baby-sitter who had put him down for his nap]?" Ben also recited letters from the names on cars, and then said the name. Such incidents reassured me that Ben was progressing, but at his own pace.

Ben returned for the second year of the same program at school in the fall of 1992, but the school's structure and physical plan had been drastically changed over the summer. Instead of 10 students and two instructors, now there were almost 20 students to two staff. Some students attended for the entire day, others, like Ben, just for the morning. The class was moved to a larger room. Ben did not learn the other children's names this time and seldom acknowledged their presence. He found his old puzzles and continued taking them apart and putting them together. Although some new items attracted his interest, such as painting with watercolors on an easel, he seemed to be aimlessly wandering around the room a great deal of the time when I observed him. One day in the fall, he enthusiastically greeted me and took me by the hand to see a pumpkin-shaped basket filled with small Halloween trinkets: a black cat, a ghost made of tissue, and a plastic skeleton. He took them out one at a time, naming each one as he handed it to me. Again, I was reassured.

I blamed Ben's disconnectedness and lack of attention on the larger class size and the fact the children were arriving and leaving at different times. I attended several meetings with the school administrators and other discontented parents. Several months into the school year, however, Ben's teacher indicated that she had serious concerns about Ben. For the second time she suggested that Ben start speech therapy. She wondered if he had lost his hearing; he did not respond to his name when he was called. She also mentioned that he did not make eye contact with people at school. She suggested that I contact Easter Seals for a screening. Notably, my pediatrician did not think speech therapy was required as long as Ben was learning new words. Nonetheless, I set up a screening with the school district for December.

In December, shortly after his third birthday, Ben was screened by the school district to determine if he met the criterion for admission into the Developmental Preschool Program—6 months' delay in development. Conducting the evaluation were a special education teacher, Christie, and a speech therapist, Cathy. Ben marched in happily, noticed the life-sized Santa Claus in a rocking chair, and repeated "Santa" several times. Later, when he saw a picture of a dog, he said "dog" over and over. While the two women were evaluating Ben, I filled out a questionnaire in an office. My heart sank as I read the questions: Except for his ability with puzzles, Ben had accomplished very few of the milestones a 3-year-old should.

Christie and Cathy explained that although Ben did not complete the screening because he could not follow their directions, they did observe him perform many of the tasks for which they were testing as he went about the room playing. They mentioned that his speech was "perseverative" and that he was not generating his own sentences. I agreed. His sentences were limited to quotations taken from characters in books or videos. We used to read stories to Ben, and were amazed that he could recite these verbatim. I remembered handing him a toy, and he said, " 'How nice, said Lowly Worm.' " This was a direct quote from a Richard Scarry book. When I asked what could cause perseverative speech, they responded that the cause could be neurological. They recommended that the school district order comprehensive tests for Ben.

I telephoned the pediatrician as soon as we got home. He was very surprised Ben did not pass the screening. I told him that the speech therapist said Ben's perseverative speech could be caused by a neurological problem. He suggested we see the pediatric neurologist who had diagnosed Ben's facial asymmetry when crying. I was able to make an appointment for the following day.

The appointment with the neurologist, Dr. Eugene Schnitzler, did not go well. Ben seemed more restless than usual, circling the room and touching everything. He would not show the doctor how well he could put together the puzzle I had brought. The doctor tried, unsuccessfully, to get a response from Ben when he called his name. He checked Ben's reflexes and then handed the little hammer to Ben. Ben took it and placed it against his cheek.

The neurologist told me Ben had Pervasive Developmental Disorder (PDD), a "garbage can" diagnosis ascribed to children who were developing abnormally without a known cause. I never heard of such a diagnosis. I asked if Ben would recover. Some children did recover, he answered, but for most it was a lifelong disability. "How upset should I be?" I asked. "It's quite serious," he said. I asked how I could help Ben. He told me to contact the school district and they would "take care" of us. He added that he expected I would remember very little of what he had said and surmised he would be hearing from my husband with further questions. We could get a blood test for fragile X syndrome and an EEG, but he expected they would be normal (they were). The appointment over, we left.

I called Abe as soon as I returned home. He immediately called the neurologist, who used the word *autism* for the first time to describe Ben's condition. Abe continued to see patients for the rest of the afternoon, came home in the evening, and burst into tears. Ben watched as Abe cried and began to cry too. I still had not, and would not, for several days. "He would be better off dead," Abe sobbed. But Ben did not seem autistic to me.

The pediatrician called that night. "Ben's autistic," he said. "You should see Dr. Leventhal at the University of Chicago." I didn't sleep that night. I wanted to see Dr. Leventhal.

The next morning I called Dr. Bennett Leventhal's office. He wasn't seeing new patients. I called a psychiatrist I knew who was a graduate of University of Chicago to ask if he could arrange an appointment as a favor. Instead, he recommended that I call a friend of his, an expert on language disorders who had worked with and evaluated disabled children for many years, Bonnie Litowitz, Ph.D.

I phoned Dr. Litowitz immediately. She listened carefully, and asked a few questions: "Does Ben rock?" "Yes, in his rocking chair while he watches television." "Does Ben have tantrums?" "Never." She said she would come and observe Ben at school and advise us. I believed she thought the neurologist might have been mistaken. Finally, I could cry.

I told Ben's teacher that Dr. Litowitz would be coming to observe Ben and that the neurologist told us Ben was autistic. "Does that mean he's really smart?" she asked. I wasn't sure what it meant. A stop at the library was in order. Much of what was described in one book on autism did not ring true for Ben—he wasn't hyperactive; he was a marvelous eater, not picky at all; he wasn't retarded. But I was startled to read over and over that the children were "beautiful." That described Ben. I looked up "Autism" in the phone book and left a message on the answering machine at the State Autism Society.

After observing Ben at school, Dr. Litowitz came home with him and Abe. As they walked in the door, Ben slipped, fell hard, and cried. He reached up for me and I soothed him in my lap. After lunch together, Dr. Litowitz said the words I had been praying to hear: "Ben is not autistic." She had seen a boy like Ben before. She thought he had speech and social delay, but this could be helped by speech and play therapy. We would begin speech therapy after New Year's Day. She would help us locate a therapist. I knew her evaluation had to be more accurate than the neurologist's. He had observed Ben so briefly, and in a strange environment.

The staff person at the Autism Society returned my call. She found it incredulous that Dr. Schnitzler could have made a mistake, and seemed to mistrust Dr. Litowitz's analysis. As I certainly did not want to learn about autism if I did not have to, I decided not to join the organization.

Ben began his twice-weekly sessions with speech therapist Pat Van Slyke in January. She too questioned the PDD/autistic label because Ben had a great deal of speech and "seems intelligent." The initial evaluation went quite well. He was able to label body parts, and labeled pictures when I cued him by saying, "It's a _____." At Pat's request, he gave a teddy bear a drink. His functional expressive language was estimated at 18–24 months. She instructed us to require a verbalization from Ben, like "want juice," before catering to his needs. Ben did begin demanding candy, cookies, and television after just a few sessions. Whereas his functional language started to improve, other idiosyncratic behaviors appeared. He began sucking on two fingers almost constantly. He started to drop his cup or spoon more frequently, and would not get down from his chair to retrieve them as he had in the past. It was as if they disappeared for him once they were out of sight. Dr. Litowitz thought the finger sucking might be from anxiety as we began to demand more of Ben.

Ben changed preschools to another Montessori one with only six children, all younger than he. The instructor happened to be a speech therapist. Sometimes after school I would wander into an empty classroom designed for older children and Ben would play with some of the early reading materials. He was still especially interested in the alphabet and would spell out car names seen as he passed through the parking lot—"T-O-Y-O-T-A"—or "W-E-L-C-O-M-E" on a welcome mat. Dr. Seuss was a favorite and he memorized many of his books, which he would gleefully recite at family gatherings.

The evaluations from the school district were scheduled. The hearing test was difficult to administer because Ben would not follow directions. However, he turned toward the sound of a mechanical bear playing the drums and the audiologist thought he could hear. The psychological evaluation showed Ben's level of cognitive development to be that of a 17-month-old. His skills were "widely scattered," meaning he experienced difficulty with many early tasks while correctly performing many of the more complicated ones. His strongest skills were in the area of visual discrimination, nonverbal reasoning, and problem solving. He performed board tasks higher than the 30-month age level. His written language skills were rated at 4 years 2 months. The psychologist administered the Childhood Autism Rating Scale (CARS) and noted that Ben's functioning in three areas were rated as being within normal limits: adaptation to change, anxiety reactions, and activity level. During the evaluation, Ben adapted to changes readily and displayed no desire for sameness. He found it difficult, though, to remain seated and wandered the room unless he was physically prompted to remain seated.

The multidisciplinary conference with the school district was quite upsetting. Dr. Litowitz was concerned because the psychologist and the school representatives seemed to be more focused on behavior management issues, whereas she thought Ben's strengths—academics—should be the concern.

Ben started attending the developmental preschool in March. It was a 3-hour program Tuesday through Friday. The Montessori program allowed him to continue on Mondays. He began to wander continuously unless he was "reading" a book, reciting a memorized story, or eating a snack. His eye contact was very poor but improved after about a month in the new classroom. He never seemed upset and would sit in his teacher's lap, spontaneously giving her hugs.

After 11 sessions of the twice weekly speech therapy, Pat noticed Ben was demonstrating fully emerging interaction and mutual engagement with her. He was beginning to understand taking turns and playing with Pat and repeated "all done" when each activity ended.

That spring, I enrolled Ben in Tumbling Tots at the park district, a six-session, half-hour class. I thought he would enjoy the activity and that the exposure to typical children his age would do him good. Unfortunately, there was only one instructor for seven 3-year-old children. Because Ben could not stay seated or do tasks without physical assistance, the instructor asked that we not continue.

I believed that Ben should be enrolled in more activities during the day. Except for television, he could not entertain himself nor be entertained by any sedentary activity such as board games. Although Pat demonstrated some activities Ben enjoyed, such as watching her blow bubbles and listening to songs and nursery rhymes, I needed to hold Ben in my lap to keep him from wandering no matter how enjoyable he found the activity. He had no sense of danger and could not be left alone. He began chewing on the cuffs of his sleeves and the collars of his shirts. We took long walks, shopped, went to the playground, and ran errands. I found an early childhood swim program that required that a parent stay with the child in the water. Because it was held in the evenings, Abe took Ben to this activity. Ben showed no fear of the water and was able to participate fully.

Ben also took a weekly, half-hour Kindermusik class, which initially also required a parent to be present. I would help Ben stay seated in my lap on the floor or guide him for the group activities. We repeated this class for three sessions until he got too old to have a parent present.

We took Ben to a family gathering in Los Angeles. He went through the Disneyland attractions and seemed to enjoy them all, especially a live performance of "Beauty and the Beast."

When we got home, we replaced the crib in Ben's room with a regular bed. He adjusted immediately and we had no problem with him wandering around after putting him to bed.

In general, I was pleased with the progress Ben was making in school and therapy. The notes sent home from school were upbeat about Ben's eye contact and language. Despite this, I remained uneasy because he had not regained his ability to concentrate on a project or any of the socialization skills he had 12 months earlier.

As summer approached, we learned about a day camp in Skokie near where I had grown up and our parents lived, run by Keshet, an organization for Jewish children with disabilities. Children with disabilities were assigned an aide and participated fully with typical peers in a

Jewish Community Center-sponsored camp. I would have to drive 40 miles each way to take Ben there, but we stayed overnight with family one or two nights a week. As the school district summer program lasted only half of the summer, I decided to take Ben to camp two days a week until summer school was over, then full time in July and August.

There was not an aide for Ben the first week of the district summer school; it was disappointing to see him wandering around the classroom. However, he started drinking from a straw for the first time. Now I could give Ben juice boxes to take to camp and to drink on the long car ride there.

We started private occupational therapy once a week, as we thought it would reduce Ben's mouthing of objects. The therapist recommended brushing him every 2 hours with a soft surgical brush: quick brush strokes on the back, arms, palms, legs, and soles of his feet, followed by joint compressions. He enjoyed it when she swung him in a rope hammock and wrapped him in a blanket. Regrettably, we did not notice any improvement in mouthing. We continued with speech therapy with Pat, but on a weekly basis, as she took time off.

I was pleased with the Keshet camp. Ben's aide was an undergraduate in special education and was well supervised by a certified special education teacher. There were 5 developmentally disabled children in the group of 17 children. The head counselor's attitude toward Ben and the other Keshet children could not have been more welcoming. She had observed that the typical children benefited from the experience by learning tolerance and consideration. Ben needed full assistance with the crafts but was showing improvement in swimming with the daily practice.

As long as Ben and I were staying overnight in the northern suburbs, Dr. Litowitz suggested that Ben might enjoy a weekly half-hour of music therapy at the Institute for Therapy Through the Arts in Glencoe. After the first few sessions, Ben's therapist, Joanie, had created a very pleasant interlude in his day. Using a very structured approach, she started by singing a short welcoming song accompanied by the guitar. She made picture cards of nursery rhymes and some of Ben's favorite songs and let Ben choose by pointing which ones he wanted to hear. She gently prodded him to beat a drum, strum her guitar, and push a few keys on the piano. At the close of class, she ended with the "I Love You" theme from *Barney*.

By the end of the summer, however, Ben's speech had diminished. He could no longer count and seemed unable to recite books he had memorized. Remaining only was his ability to fill in the last word of a phrase. He seemed to have trouble "finding" the word he wanted to say and would draw out the sounds. Pat was not particularly concerned with the loss of "nonfunctional" speech or Ben's delayed verbal production. She did not consider the loss of "parrotlike" language to be a regression. Although she was positive about Ben's "progress," she told me she could no longer provide therapy because she was returning to school. My sister recommended an interim therapist in Evanston while I searched for a new one closer to home. Dr. Litowitz had no suggestions.

The interim therapist was very concerned about the losses in Ben's speech. She suggested I see Dr. Joseph Pasternak at Evanston Hospital, a pediatric neurologist whom she found to be very thorough.

Dr. Pasternak ordered an extensive evaluation. Ben had a retinal examination by an ophthalmologist. He also had an MRI scan and a second EEG. Results of a metabolic workup, including a complete blood count, electrolytes, liver, thyroid, and kidney tests, biotinidase, acylcarnitine profile, urine organic acids, urine amino acids, and blood amino acids, were all normal. The fragile X assay result was also normal. Abe and I took Ben to a geneticist who took skin from Ben's arm for fibroblast testing. He tested for galactosidase, beta-mannosidase, hexosaminidase-A, arylsulfatase-A, and galactocerebrosidase. All test results were normal. This ruled out GM-1 gangliosidosis, beta-mannosidosis, Tay–Sachs disease and its variants, metachromatic leukodystrophy, and Krabbe's disease.

Ben returned to the Geneva Developmental Preschool in the fall of 1993. He had his own one-to-one aide to help him stay focused with class activities. A typical day for Ben included: (1) leaving the bus and walking to the classroom, (2) working on taking off his coat and backpack and hanging them up (with pictures to identify activities), (3) sitting at circle time, (4) participating in free play and sensorimotor activities (some of which he could choose by picture or object; others he had to complete), (5) sitting and participating in music, (6) sitting and participating in snack time, (7) participating in gross motor activities, (8) participating in sensorimotor activities, (9) putting on his coat, and (10) walking to the bus. Ben sat at circle time with varying success.

Some days he would find his own picture and put it on a felt board to indicate he was present. All art projects needed to be done with hand-over-hand assistance. He had individual occupational therapy, involving rolling on balls and scooter boards. His teachers worked on getting Ben to extend his arms and push himself off the floor. They also had some success with roller skating. Cathy Reynolds, a speech therapist, was in the classroom, but despite her efforts to keep Ben talking, he continued to lose his memorized nursery rhymes and songs. He was still, however, asking for his snack.

On Ben's return to school, his teachers remarked how limp he had become walking down stairs. Abe believed this was related to Ben's need to seek out uneven or moving surfaces to stand on so he could lose and regain his balance. We encouraged his teachers to "be brave" and let Ben solo down the stairs. We assured them that if they were not there to support him he could go downstairs independently, as he had been doing for years at home.

Ben was enrolled in various after-school activities in the fall of 1993. He had a half-hour of individual tumbling and movement through our special recreation association with Tracey Weinum. Tracey was very warm and enthusiastic, and gave Ben much encouragement as he walked the balance beam, jumped on the minitramp, and worked on somersaults and forward rolls. She also was the inclusion specialist for the association. I asked for her help in enrolling Ben in Tumbling Tots at the Geneva Park District after school. Previously, I had explained to the park district curriculum supervisor that Ben still could not follow verbal directions, and requested to stay with Ben during the class to guide him through. The supervisor was insistent that parents were not allowed because separation from parents was a goal of the program. Tracey told me that besides making physical changes to the park district building, the district was required by the Americans with Disabilities Act to make a "reasonable accommodation" to allow participation of disabled children in scheduled activities. After she talked to the curriculum supervisor, he called me to say the park district would provide an aide at the district's expense. Ben was admitted to the tumbling program, and although his tumbling skills waxed and waned during the several sessions he was enrolled, I received great satisfaction knowing that the park district had received an education about their obligation to children with special needs in the district.

Shortly after Ben's fourth birthday, I found a new speech therapist who would work with Ben once each week at our home. Our weekly visits to Evanston came to an end. Amy Engdahl came with a laptop computer and, after weeks of prompting, Ben started using a jellybean switch to "turn the page" of simple stories and songs on a CD-ROM. Amy also had Ben use switches to activate battery-powered animals and toys. I appreciated her efforts to motivate Ben, who was getting more and more difficult to reach. Because he still said a few words, mostly parroting the name of a snack food, I was surprised when she began constructing picture cards of fruits and other snack foods so Ben could point to what he wanted. She suggested this as a way for Ben to make choices, rather than to just take or leave what I offered.

I tried to get Cathy, the classroom speech therapist, to observe what Amy was doing with the computer, but she had no interest. It disappointed me that she was not interested in the latest methods to teach children like Ben.

Around this time, friends and relatives began bringing articles about Catherine Maurice's book, *Let Me Hear Your Voice,* to my attention. The book gave an account of an autistic child's successful experience with an extensive behavior modification program employed at UCLA by Dr. Ivor Lovaas. Testimonials to this method appeared more and more frequently in the autism newsletters to which we subscribed. We learned by calling UCLA that their graduate students would supervise a Lovaas program for Ben if we could find college students to implement it. I called some local colleges and asked to speak with the department chairs in psychology. The professor at Wheaton College said his department was already involved in a similar program coordinated by a UCLA Ph.D., Dr. Anne Maxwell, who was living in Chicago. He gave me her phone number.

Dr. Maxwell explained how her program worked. She would run a weekend workshop on the behavior modification techniques at our home for the student therapists, our family, and school personnel interested in attending. Therapy could be done after school and on weekends. She would help us recruit the student therapists from local colleges. Before we began therapy, another psychologist, Joyce Hopkins, would test Ben to establish a baseline. Dr. Maxwell would come to our home every 2 weeks for 2 hours to meet with the therapists, answer their questions, observe them working with Ben, and demonstrate the proper techniques. We would pay Dr. Maxwell $1500 for the weekend program, $200 for the bimonthly visits, and the students $10 an hour for the 20 hours of therapy per week.

I took Ben for his baseline assessment in October 1993. Ben wandered the room incessantly and Dr. Hopkins was unable to test Ben on any of the structured activities on the Bayley test. Nonetheless, she advised me to start looking for a conventional preschool for the following fall, because by that time Ben would surely be ready to participate. Although it was hard to imagine, especially considering Ben's behavior during the assessment, it felt good to hear positive things about Ben and to feel hopeful again. I was also intrigued by the thought of him using his free time in a constructive way.

With Dr. Maxwell's input, we assembled a team of four student therapists. Two were graduate students in psychology, one at Wheaton College and the other working toward a Ph.D. at Illinois Institute of Technology under Dr. Hopkins. The third was a Wheaton College graduate with a degree in early childhood education, taking time off before returning to a masters' program, and the fourth, a high school graduate, was Ben's aide at school.

Dr. Maxwell presented her training for the therapists over a weekend in November 1993. Using a discrete trial format, the students would drill Ben to "Look at me," "Come here," and "Sit down." Once these were mastered, Ben would be ready to learn. Christie, Ben's developmental preschool teacher, attended and agreed to support the effort.

While we were setting up the Lovaas program at home for Ben, his preschool was looking for guidance. Ben wasn't progressing toward the goals set at the multidisciplinary conference. The school consulted another speech therapist, Jenny Potonos, from Krejci Academy, a school for autistic children in Naperville, a neighboring suburb. She observed Ben at school and came to our home to observe while a student therapist worked with Ben. She was disturbed by the drill using juice and a snack because only a verbalized request was rewarded, even though she observed Ben communicating nonverbally that he wanted a drink or a bite. Jenny believed that pointing to a picture would constitute a better drill. She was afraid that we were "extinguishing" Ben's efforts to communicate by forcing him to speak. In addition, she suggested the school prepare daily picture schedule/choice boards, paired with verbalizations and written words. For transitioning, she made small signs indicating start and stop. She also suggested taking one or two activities—such as requiring him to help with dressing and clearing his plate from the table—from the behavior modification program we were using at home and requiring Ben complete them at school, but letting him have a choice of activities at other times. She thought the classroom should accept a gaze as indicating a choice.

I voiced my concern to Jenny that Ben still seemed to be losing skills in the early childhood special education program. I had also begun hearing that the preschool program for 1994–1995 was going to change to an inclusion program with the Geneva Park District Preschool. Classes were going to be held only three mornings each week, instead of the current four. She suggested that I obtain an evaluation and educational consultation from Dr. Marjorie Getz, a woman with a doctorate in special education, who had been able to help various families obtain appropriate services and programming for their children. I gave her office a call and made the earliest available appointment in May.

Abe and I took Ben to Miami Beach for a week's vacation in January 1994. He was calm and relaxed for the flight and seemed to enjoy the break from the winter weather. We took him through the Everglades and although he never focused on any of the birds or reptiles, he stayed on the boardwalks with no trouble. We also took a ride on a glass-bottomed boat in the Keys. As long as we strolled around the cabin occasionally, he did not seem to have any trouble adjusting to the new activities.

The student therapists were diligent and stuck to their schedules throughout the winter. Ben received the behavior modification training 20 hours a week Monday through Saturday, some of it in school. Potty training was included as one of the drills, accompanied by undressing and dressing. Ben was taken to the bathroom on a schedule, or when he began to wet himself. He still had no way of indicating when he needed to go. The Lovaas therapy continued over 10 months, costing over $10,000. In retrospect, Ben received no lasting benefit.

Dr. Getz came out to observe Ben at school and interviewed Abe and me at our home. She also had Ben come to her office in May for a cognitive evaluation. Unlike Dr. Hopkins, who allowed Ben to wander about her office, Dr. Getz placed Ben in a highchair to complete the Bayley Scale of Infant Development and the CARS when he got wiggly. She was able to get a score. The results horrified me; his age equivalent was 7 months! On the Child Development Inventory, the results were as follows:

Subscales	Current score	Age at which skills were achieved and lost
Social	12 months	16 months
Self-help	14.5 months	20 months
Gross motor	23 months	2 years
Fine motor	17 months	18 months
Expressive language	13 months	2 years 2 months
Language comprehension	<12 months	16 months
Letters	2 years	3 years 4 months
Numbers	18 months	2 years 4 months
General development	16 months	21 months

I had thought that the intensive programs we had put Ben through would have at least halted his regression. Everything I had read about autism lauded early intervention. It was tremendously frightening to learn that Ben's impairment was severe and progressive. I made an appointment for Ben to see Dr. Leventhal at the University of Chicago in June.

Dr. Getz accompanied us to Ben's IEP meeting at the end of the school year. Both the classroom teacher, Christie, and the speech therapist, Cathy, observed that Ben's basic single-word and occasional two-word phrases had disappeared. Cathy reported observing "search behaviors" when Ben was attempting to communicate. He would repeat the initial consonant of a word, denoting an attempt to say it, but was unable to complete the word. Christie believed that Ben's ability to sit and attend had increased over the year, but his ability to do tasks fluctuated. They also noted there were some things Ben could do in the fall that he could no longer do. I had anticipated a recommendation that Ben continue the three mornings per week inclusion program. Although I feared hurting Christie's feelings, I believed that Ben needed more classroom activity, and I needed Ben to attend school more often. Unless he was under close supervision, Ben continued to wander around the house or circle the television. He could no longer entertain himself for even a moment. Dr. Getz, a strong believer in inclusion, suggested Ben attend Krejci Academy the two days he was not in the Geneva inclusion program as well as the afternoons the inclusion preschool was in session. It sounded like it might work. In the meantime, Krejci would accept Ben into the summer school, five days a week from 9 AM until 2 PM. The summer school teacher, Marilyn Mason, taught the same class in the fall. The continuity sounded good.

Abe and I went to the University of Chicago to meet with Dr. Catherine Lord, a psychologist, as a precursor to her and Dr. Leventhal's meeting with Ben. She was genuine and warm; we liked her immediately. On a stifling hot June 15, we brought Ben to be tested. Dr. Lord believed several aspects of Ben's behavior were remarkable. One was that he seemed relatively uninterested in objects. She noticed that when no one was directing his behavior, he would wander from place to place, stopping to hug Abe or me. She observed that if someone directed his attention to an object, he would try to do something with it, but would have difficulty in sustaining his attention for more than a few seconds.

Dr. Lord found it remarkable that when Ben was presented with a task that was familiar to him, such as stacking blocks or placing objects in a container, he would start the task but become distracted by sights or sounds or some other thought and could not complete the action. For example, Ben would start to put an object in a container, and then seem to forget what he was doing and drop it or put it elsewhere. He also had difficulty releasing objects, such as when she had him put dowels in a container. As was typical of his behavior at the time, he put many of the objects in his mouth.

During the examination, Ben enjoyed hearing Dr. Lord sing, and he stood and watched her blow bubbles. She remarked how he gave such nice, clear hugs, and how tolerant he was of her attempts to get him to do things.

A variety of different instruments were used to attempt to determine Ben's developmental level. On the Mullen Scale of Early Development, Ben received an age-equivalent score of 12 months. He attained a similar result on the test of fine motor skills. On the receptive and expressive language scale, he received an age equivalent of 4 months. The same score was given on the Bayley Scale of Infant Development, with his highest marks given for turning the pages of a book and putting cubes in a cup. Other high marks included ringing a bell and looking at pages in a book. Ben had the greatest difficulty with social items, including recognition of parents, smiling when the examiner spoke (although he was observed to smile at me spontaneously), smiling in response to the examiner's smile, and vocalizing a variety of different sounds. Most of the vocalizations he did make had to do with jumping up and down and flapping his arms when he was excited, which Dr. Lord believed were not intended for communication.

After Dr. Lord finished, Dr. Leventhal performed a physical examination of Ben. His conclusions were that Ben's systems were basically normal except for marked deficits in gross and fine motor skills. Dr. Leventhal was reputed to be the most knowledgeable in the Chicago area about autism in all of its forms. I felt that if there were any breakthroughs in the field, he would be one of the first to know. I also knew that he and Dr. Lord were frequently out of the office, presenting papers and attending conferences, not only nationally, but internationally. They assured me that they would talk to other physicians and psychologists about Ben.

At this time I was 9 months pregnant with our second child. That night, I woke up in labor and we went to the hospital. Our daughter, Lea, was born several hours later. After our afternoon at the University of Chicago, I welcomed the distraction from my fears for Ben. The physical pain from labor seemed minor in comparison.

Ben started summer school at Krejci the following week. Abe, Lea, and I drove him to his first day of school. We met his teacher, Marilyn Mason, and his aide, a college student named Fred. The school, a former college dormitory built over 50 years ago, was not impressive. Ben's classroom was tiny and cramped. Nevertheless, I took an immediate liking to Marilyn. Her demeanor corroborated the assurances of Drs. Lord and Leventhal that she was a good teacher. From the first days she tried to address bothersome issues such as Ben's need to chew. When rubber tubing around his neck didn't do the trick, she found that Ben preferred a soft plastic teether. In addition to physical education, they went swimming outdoors every day. With a 5-day school week, the class had more time to go into the community than did the Geneva Developmental Preschool. They went to the grocery store to shop for their lunch items on Fridays, and took other frequent field trips.

On most days after school Ben had at least a few hours of Lovaas behavior therapy. Coordinating the self-care and cognitive drills the student therapists were doing with Marilyn's classroom activities required more effort than I would have wished. Eventually, Marilyn and Fred came by to watch an hour of the drills and left promising to be consistent when working on the same tasks. Marilyn even found a quiet private room at school for Fred and Ben to work on drills during school hours.

Over the summer Ben began to have trouble sleeping through the night. The extra swimming may have worn him out, and the long bus ride home usually put him to sleep. He would race around his room for a couple of hours each night, and wake up early, 4 or 5 in the morning.

In August, Abe took Ben back to the University of Chicago for a reevaluation. Although Ben would not or could not complete several items on the same skills inventory that he had in June, Drs. Lord and Leventhal believed that there was no major regression. They suggested that Ben stay at Krejci for the fall. So he did.

By the end of the summer, little progress had been made with the Lovaas therapy. All of the student therapists either wanted to try working with a more typically autistic child, or simply needed to get on with other activities and interests. Although I could understand their reasons for leaving, I felt abandoned by Dr. Maxwell, who was offering the therapists positions with other families before she found any replacements for us. I spoke to her about this, but she never did find new therapists for us. After the final meeting with the therapists, she never called or contacted us in any way. Considering the bright future Dr. Hopkins had predicted, Ben's tiny gains in self-care, such as bringing his plate to the sink when he had finished eating, seemed inconsequential in light of the effort and dollars poured into his training.

I placed an ad in the job postings at three area high schools. After much thought, I decided to describe Ben as "disabled." The ad solicited someone to watch Ben in the afternoons, and take him to his tumbling and swimming lessons, walks, and other activities. One school indicated they would post the ad on the condition that the language describing Ben as disabled was removed; I'm not sure why. Only one student responded, but she was wonderful: affectionate, patient, and physically strong. Sara Lindstrom answered the ad because she wanted to work with a disabled child. Shortly after she started, I learned the

YWCA in Aurora, about a 15-minute drive, had open swim for school-age children for an hour after school every day. Sara, a trained lifeguard, was the perfect companion. Within months Ben was paddling independently with no flotation devices.

Ben happily returned to Marilyn's classroom in September 1994. His program included a group music class, and individual occupational, intrusion, and speech therapy. The speech therapy consisted mainly of oral–motor exercises to prevent mouthing. In intrusion therapy, sensory awareness of tactual–kinesthetic stimuli was stressed. Textured material, weighted bags, and bags of different temperatures were placed on different parts of Ben's body. Ben enjoyed cool bags more than warm, and liked the vibrator most of all. The therapist also stressed sensory awareness of auditory stimuli. Ben showed little awareness of sound except to locate a piece of candy in a cup. Visually, he would search for a piece of candy in a light box and could locate various objects of interest to him when seated in front of a mirror.

The goal for Ben in occupational therapy was to achieve greater functional use of his hands. The therapist successfully taught Ben to propel himself with his hands in a net swing, but when she tried to get him to place bean bags in a container, he would bring them to his mouth. Instead of propelling himself on a scooter board with his hands in the prone position, Ben sought to stand on the scooter board. He also chose to stand on the rocking platform. She concluded that he sought out vestibular sensations, particularly those achieved by standing on uneven or moving surfaces and losing and recapturing his balance. I agreed this was consistent with his attraction to escalators. He had to be guarded as we passed an escalator, regardless of the direction the stairs were moving. At home, he loved to walk on toys he had dropped on the floor. However, he never stepped on the baby.

October brought Ben's fifth birthday and a week or so of crying spells. It was very unusual for Ben to cry and it disturbed us to see him unhappy. The pediatrician could not find anything wrong; the episodes remained a mystery. Ben sometimes napped at school and also on the bus going home. Most nights he could not fall asleep until 11 PM. He continued to awaken between midnight and 4 or 5 AM. Sleeping problems were the focus of our next visit to Dr. Lord in November. We discussed medication, but decided that this would not keep him from waking early, which we considered the more serious problem. Dr. Lord suggested that Ben be prevented from dozing and that he be given caffeine beverages, such as sweetened ice tea at meals and snacks, to keep him up on the bus ride home. She also recommended we increase aerobic activity and find a teether with a hole in the middle that could be strung around his neck. A teether in the shape of a hand or foot with a hole for the string became Ben's trademark accessory.

On the Bayley Scales, Ben received a raw score that was four points lower than his score in August and six points lower than his score in June. Dr. Lord did not notice a dramatic behavior change, but commented that it was much more difficult to get Ben to do anything with his hands because he was so engrossed with putting things in his mouth. He was still able to turn the pages of a book and put a cube in a cup (while holding another cube in his mouth). We were all disappointed to learn that Ben had not made progress over the summer and fall, despite the more intensive program at Krejci.

Marilyn was extremely cooperative in enforcing the nonsleep policy. An aide walked Ben outside when he seemed sleepy and found a variety of soft toys for him to bring to his mouth. The speech therapist increased the amount of oral stimulation to 5 minutes every half-hour, but Ben still sought out things to put in his mouth.

Weekends began to become very routine, consisting of Lea's need to nap and Ben's need for activity. I usually hired a sitter to take Ben for a walk in the forest preserve or to a playground, an amusement park, or an indoor play area on Saturday mornings. After lunch, Abe would take him swimming at an indoor pool, followed by a walk through the mall and dinner out. We found restaurants with highchairs and tile floors that welcomed families. Sundays the grandparents came to visit. Ben usually had an afternoon swim on that day, too. A video always played before and between activities. For special treats, we found that Ben sat well through live Disney on Ice performances, perhaps because he was so familiar with the music from his videos. He seemed to enjoy children's concerts when the performers stuck to classic songs.

In February 1995, Dr. Leventhal decided to try a course of Zoloft to deal with Ben's need for constant motion and mouthing and sleep problems. After a few weeks, Ben was taking 150 mg a day. His first nights on Zoloft, we noticed increased hyperactivity. After a week or two, that subsided but there was no noticeable improvement in Ben's mouthing, attending, or sleeping. He seemed more flat emotionally. After 3 months, we stopped the medication. The trouble with settling down for sleep at night and with early morning awakening, though, occurred in cycles that seemed to have no cause.

With the new baby, Ben's daily school commitment, my part-time job, and Sara's help after school, the weeks flew by. I still mourned for the "lost" Ben, but felt less urgency to seek out new treatments. I had learned about the Carl Pfeiffer Treatment Center in Naperville from Jenny Fairthorne, who had indicated that her husband had been in contact with them regarding their son, David. The center treated various behaviors biochemically with vitamin and mineral supplements. Drs. Leventhal and Lord thought these would not be of benefit to Ben. I eventually decided to try anyway and had Ben tested in February.

The report showed Ben had several imbalances: high histamine, hypoglycemia, zinc deficiency, and mild pyroluria. We received boxes of vitamins and minerals to give to him, including some giant capsules and tablets. He needed to take vitamins A, B_6, C, and E, pyridoxal-5-phosphate, dimethylamino ethanol-H3, chromium, calcium, magnesium, zinc, manganese, and methionine. Before bedtime, he was to take inositol. I realized he could never swallow them, and he would not finish the milk shakes designed to mask the flavor of the supplements. I called the center for suggestions and they gave me the number of a Maryland pharmacy that would consolidate the vitamins into several capsules. But that would still not solve the problem of swallowing capsules. I spoke to the pharmacist about making an elixir with a syrup, but he admitted the syrup would not hide the flavor of the supplements. I eventually just put the boxes in a closet and gave up.

Jenny Fairthorne had mentioned that David enjoyed horseback riding. I inquired about lessons at our special recreation district office. Ben had been on pony rides at a children's amusement park and tended to slide off after a few seconds. Nevertheless, I thought it would be appropriate for him to try because he was so fearless when it came to new activities and it would be a constructive use of his time after school.

The organization we found to help Ben was Friends for Therapeutic Equine Activities. Two instructors and a team of volunteer aides conduct riding lessons for disabled children and adults. They had some openings for weekly, 45-minute sessions after school at a stable not far from Ben's school. For the first lesson, three volunteer aides walked with Ben—one on either side and one to lead the horse. One of two staff members directed the aides, instructing them and the horse—a full-size animal, not a pony—to walk faster or slower. The instructor watched for Ben to become restless, and then had the horse walk faster. She theorized that Ben craved stimulation and would stay in the saddle as long as he got enough. Ben enjoyed the sensation and the experience. He never seemed frightened and more than once even fell asleep in the saddle. Other days he was very hyperactive, with lots of vocalizations and hand-flapping. At times, the instructor sat Ben facing the rear of the horse. Sometimes she removed the saddle so that Ben could ride lying down.

Riding gave us an entertaining destination for all but the coldest months of the year. It was not easy to find places to take Ben where he was engaged in something constructive and fun and where he felt welcome and accepted. Rain or shine, freezing or hot, Ben got the exercise and activity he craved in a structured and safe environment. After the disappointment with tumbling, it was wonderful to see Ben acquiring new skills and concentrating on this sport in addition to swimming. Soon he began riding twice weekly.

The Krejci staff and I met in the spring of 1995 to discuss Ben's progress and plan for summer and fall. The report was similar to that of the Geneva Developmental Preschool in 1993 and 1994, noting that after months of practice, Ben was sitting for longer periods of time with the group and reaching for his photo at circle time as long as his was the last one on the board. Using his utensils to eat continued to be a problem. Although his participation in oral stimulation, sensory stimulation, and behavior training programs was highly inconsistent, they observed that the one activity he attended to consistently was watching videos. Toileting was also inconsistent. We decided to call Dr. Lord to provide programming suggestions.

Dr. Lord suggested the following activities as appropriate for Ben: (1) putting things in containers, (2) teaming several actions together prior to receiving a small piece of food (e.g., pulling a string to get a pretzel, unwrapping a piece of food, moving a cup to see what was underneath), and (3) tickling, clapping, touching, and similar physical routines. The latter activities were intended to evoke an anticipatory response and perhaps encourage Ben to move toward somebody, tolerate touching, or make eye contact. This could provide structure in his social interactions. She also suggested taking Ben to the toilet at short intervals, and then increasing the time between intervals. Another suggestion was that an obstacle course be set up in the gym for Ben to use throughout the day. Finally, she proposed keeping Ben's left hand in a felt-lined cup while he ate with his right to keep the left hand from "feeling" the food on the plate.

Ben participated in the Krejci summer school program for the second summer. His swimming skills continued to improve, and he began to explore the playground equipment more appropriately, climbing up the ladders to slide instead of trying to walk up slides, and doing less searching for objects to put in his mouth.

As Lea reached her first birthday in June, I felt a need to work with Ben not only after school but in the mornings before the school bus arrived as well. When I was alone, I was torn between attending to Ben and responding to Lea's need for my attention. As several of my friends had done, I applied to an agency for a European au pair. I specifically required an au pair candidate who had expressed an interest in working with a special needs child. The agency at first had me call candidates who had not stated an interest on their application, and I found this to be fruitless. I was afraid someone would accept the position just to get to the United States and then ask for a different host family after meeting Ben. I had to forcefully insist that I would not even consider those who had not made their preference known in their application to work with a disabled child. After a few weeks, I received an application from a 21-year-old English woman named Melanie Davies who wanted to work with a disabled child, preferably hearing impaired. I had the agency send her our application and then I spoke to her on the phone. She was hearing impaired herself. An office worker, she had no experience working with special needs children. Despite receiving several other calls, she accepted our offer. In August she arrived.

Having an au pair was very helpful because I could structure her work schedule to suit my needs. Whereas the high school baby-sitters were reliable and full of enthusiasm, they had many other activities and family commitments. Melanie, having left her old life for a year, could focus more on Ben's needs and our need to have him busy. She immediately obtained her Illinois driver's license and was able to take Ben to after-school activities, parks, and swimming. She was there on the mornings I needed help, on the school holidays, and during vacations. Another pair of hands was always welcome. Although she had no special training or experience with mentally impaired children, she did not seem to need it. We could answer most of her questions based on the advice we had been given by therapists and teachers. It was more important to us that her attitude toward Ben was cheerful and gentle. Even her hearing impairment was a plus as Ben's late-night awakenings did not disturb her sleep. She was fresh when Abe and I were exhausted from a bad night.

In the fall of 1995, I felt it was time to see another neurologist. It had been 2 years since Ben's second EEG was performed, and I was not satisfied that Landau–Kleffner had been fully explored. I asked Dr. Lord for a suggestion and she recommended that we see Dr. Meryl Lipton, a pediatric neurologist at Rush-Presbyterian–St. Luke's Hospital in Chicago.

Dr. Lipton explained that she was not an expert in Landau–Kleffner, but agreed that a sleep-deprived EEG, which had never been performed on Ben, was not a bad idea. Marilyn (who continued as Ben's teacher), Abe, and I had observed some tremors in Ben's upper body, and this was something we had never explored earlier. Dr. Lipton promised to share the results of her examination of Ben with other doctors at Rush in an attempt to deal with some of Ben's symptoms.

I found the EEG supervisor to be very helpful. When the technician had trouble attaching the wires to Ben's head, he simply wrapped Ben tightly in a sheet. This had the effect of relaxing Ben as well as immobilizing him. The EEG result was normal. Dr. Lipton suggested we return in a year for a follow-up appointment.

In the 1995–1996 school year, Ben joined a class of older girls with severe developmental delays for their music, physical education, and swimming classes. Ben now had a double dose of these classes each week. Marilyn felt the extra programming improved his ability to sit through the music class. She noticed improvement in his eye contact, facial affect, and self-help skills. Regrettably, he showed no interest in cognitive concepts such as matching, and he needed full physical assistance to complete tasks designed to teach object permanence.

A 3-year review of Ben's placement was ordered for the spring of 1996. As requested by the school district, I went to visit the self-contained classroom for our community. Clearly, it would be a bad match. The room was cheerfully cluttered with toys, various tables and chairs, and mats. Half of the eight children were nonambulatory. A brown rabbit roamed the room. The activities didn't seem appropriate for Ben (or the other children, for that matter)—the group activity of the day was Valentines, and only one child was able to do any of the work without hand-over-hand assistance. I pictured Ben stepping on the boy laying in the corner and pulling out his feeding tubes to chew on. There was no separate motor room for Ben to take a break in—he would be wandering the halls to work off energy. Although the facility offered the possibility of daily recess and weekly physical education and music with typical peers, it would come at too high a price.

At the review, the district representatives did not press the issue of moving Ben to the district's classroom. Everyone agreed that, now that Ben seemed to have stabilized, it was important to maintain his skills in an environment that specialized in dealing with his difficulties. Compared to what I had observed in the district's classroom, I felt Ben was in good hands at Krecji, but I was disappointed that, except for increased eye contact at times, very little had been accomplished. We wanted to communicate with Ben, but except for choosing between two videotapes by allowing him to touch the preferred one, no one had succeeded in creating a system we could use. Photos representing objects and activities apparently held no meaning for Ben.

We recognized that Ben's intense desire to mouth objects and his need to move around the classroom were interfering with learning. Dr. Leventhal suggested we try Ritilin to increase Ben's ability to focus. Ben started with a half of a 5 mg tablet and eventually went to three tablets a day. We kept it a secret from his teacher Marilyn for one week. When asked if there had been an improvement in Ben's level of attention, she believed there was. At home, there was little change, but we continued with the drug.

Ben was assigned to a new classroom at Krejci in the summer of 1996. He did not fit in with Marilyn's other students who had mastered their self-help needs in kindergarten and were working on academic drills. His new colleagues were all nonverbal and in diapers, like himself. Toileting and feeding, as well as frequent breaks to walk or use the playground outdoors, took up much of the schoolday.

Fall brought another new teacher to Ben's class, a new au pair— Nina Sorri of Finland—and a change of aides. I tried to maintain continuity by sending Nina to school with Ben to show how we assisted Ben at home, and asked that she watch how they did "tablework"—such as simple inset puzzles and matching—at school to carry over to home. Instead of a photo of a toilet, a laminated toilet paper roll was Velcroed to the classroom door. Ben was required to tear it off whenever he set off for a scheduled bathroom visit. It was hoped that someday he would indicate his desire to go by tearing the roll off the door. We decided to implement this at home.

Ben was still bothered by moodiness—some weeks he was so manic he could hardly sit to eat and was unable to relax to sleep, others we would find him laying on his bed with a tear running down his face for no apparent reason. We found that Depakote sprinkled on his breakfast and supper, four capsules per meal, caused an obvious improvement. Although he continued to have "ups and downs," the swings were less pronounced. The improvement in his sleep that we noted initially (but which later faded) was particularly helpful.

The 1996–1997 school year was marked by Ben's accomplishments in his recreational pursuits. At age 7, he could both ice skate and roller skate independently, so long as someone could direct him to stay moving counterclockwise. With the help of an insightful swim teacher, Mary Kay Bakken, he began to swim laps using a breaststroke—20 lengths or more—and later began surface diving to such an extent he rarely did anything else in the water. Unless he was in a bad mood, he ran, walked, and galloped along the forest trails, sometimes darting off to circle a building, jump in a puddle or other body of water (however large or small), grab a leaf to chew, or stand at a water fountain, indicating his thirst. He sat well in the saddle for most of the 45-minute horseback ride twice a week, particularly when wearing a weighted vest, and stood in his stirrups when commanded with a physical prompt by the aide. The point of all this activity was to fill the time after school and help his sleeping, but many nights—usually in bunches—nothing helped. With Dr. Leventhal's consent, we discontinued Ritilin with no apparent effect on Ben.

Over the course of a few weeks in the spring, Ben began to stay dry in his pull-up diaper for longer and longer periods. Soon, he was wearing underpants at school, then home, then in the school bus and car. Although the period after swimming and nights were still problems, a milestone that surprised and thrilled us was finally reached.

Our bubble burst late in the summer. By the start of the new school year, Ben was wetting himself so often that he had to go back to pull-ups. He was also going an entire week with trouble settling for sleep until as late as 2 AM, accompanied by waking as early as 5 in the morning. He began making loud outbursts—full-throated screams—before he slept, and other times as well. We questioned whether Nina's departure was the cause. Her replacement, our third au pair, had quit after only a few weeks, with a month of Ben's summer vacation to go. With a variety of unseasoned caregivers and harried parents, his routine was shattered, perhaps causing the cluster of negative behavior. Or perhaps it was only a coincidence.

To determine the cause of this mysterious regression, we engaged the behavior consultants at Krejci once he returned in late August 1997. Using the notebook that passed back and forth from home to school to jog my memory, I charted the date, school and home activity (antecedent), and his sleep and toileting behavior for their study. The consultants collected the papers for further review, but immediately made some helpful suggestions, such as preventing Ben from drinking fluids after 7 PM and lining his pull-up with underpants. Ben's aide and teacher attended the meeting and participated in the discussion. It felt good to discuss Ben's problems with professionals with lots of experience, even if the chart never revealed a pattern that provided an answer for us.

To this day, Ben's problems continue. As long as we have to deal with these immediate concerns, it is harder to focus on the big picture of his development, which is not too bright.

Three years have passed since Drs. Lord and Leventhal said that Ben's prognosis for a recovery of his language and cognitive skills was extremely poor. In fact, Dr. Lord suggested that if Abe and I wanted a normal home life for ourselves and Lea, Ben could not live with us beyond age 10 or 11. However, she did not know of any place, bad or good, where Ben could live other than with us. I am still processing this information. Although my feelers are out for living situations for this Ben of the future, I do not have a great desire to find out about what is available for a child with Ben's limited skills. I am afraid of what I may learn. Until it feels right, I will wait. I fear our greatest challenges are still ahead. When Ben bounces out of bed at night, who will lie down with him if we do not? I think I know the answer, and it scares me.

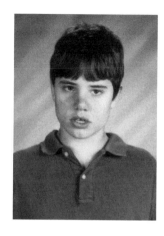

Eight

The River Jordan

by Craig Schulze

Shortly after I learned that my wife Jill was pregnant with our first child, I was sharing the news with a colleague of mine many years my senior. She smiled at my enthusiasm with grandmotherly knowing and then proceeded to launch into a protracted monologue about how all of my days from this one forward would be filled with thoughts, fears, hopes, and eventually memories of this child. Another colleague came in on the tailend of the conversation and in a pithy summary said, "Yes indeed, that first child runs through you like a river."

And so it has been: For 15 years, Jill and I have been awash in the River Jordan. Sometimes that river has been calm and beautiful; sometimes it has presented capricious twists and turns, leading to unexpected destinations; and sometimes it has raged and crashed around us, shaking the very foundations of our faith in life itself. Throughout this journey, our situation has been complicated by the fact of its sheer uniqueness. All of us know that the river of parenthood can run wild, or become polluted, or dry up. Children get sick or have accidents, behave in self-destructive ways, or even die prematurely. But rivers don't mysteriously run uphill, or form dizzying and seemingly endless eddies, or simply disappear. Children don't develop normally for 2 years and then suddenly—without evidence of brain malfunction or other apparent cause—turn into psychotic mockeries of their former selves. In 1984, however, this is precisely what happened to our son Jordan. Even in collaboration, it is unlikely that the minds of George Orwell and Rod Serling could have come up with a more peculiar and chilling tale.

Several years ago, I wrote a book called *When Snow Turns to Rain,* which chronicled my family's experiences in raising what we were told was an autistic child. Part of the motivation for writing that book was to help parents avoid the predators of the "Autism is Curable" industry that lurk around this disorder even today, but I was also interested in telling a story about a child who developed in a manner unlike any I had ever heard of or seen. Even years afterward, I was convinced that the trajectory of Jordan's life was so bizarre that it could never be repeated. That is until I began conversing with Madeline Catalano and learned of the Childhood Disintegrative Disorder (CDD) diagnosis.

The families from whom you have heard in this volume have told stories about children whose lives have been as wildly improbable as Jordan's, and reading the accounts has been an eerie experience of déjà vu. The meteoric rise and fall of these children; their slow and painful—in some cases nonexistent—paths to recovery; and the agonizing search of their parents through the educational, psychological, and medical mazes for treatment were all as I had experienced them. It was almost as if some diabolical playwright had written the script, seen it performed by my family, and then returned to it later to ask, "Now what would this be like with a family of rural New Zealanders playing the parts?"

Aside from rekindling the memories of pain, confusion, frustration, and even humor, reading these chapters has had another significant impact on me. It has verified an intuition that I have held even in my lowest moments; that is, that someday we would take the preliminary steps toward understanding what went wrong with Jordan. The diagnosis of CDD is just the beginning of a process that will subdivide the functionally useless label of autism into subgroups that can be better studied to find causes, preventive strategies, and cures.

In the previous chapters, you have read about children who are now 10 years of age or younger. Much of what they and their parents went through bears a strong resemblance to our experience with Jordan. I have therefore decided that this chapter will focus more on the period of Jordan's life between the ages of 8 and 14. A reader interested in his early development should refer to the aforementioned book *When Snow Turns to Rain.*

Jordan was born in the spring of 1982. He was slightly undersized at birth, weighing in at 6 lb 7 oz. Though fragile looking, he was free of any discernible defect other than hypospadias (crooked penis). From the beginning, he was a fairly easy baby who nursed readily, cried about an average amount, and slept through the night early on. As he grew, we noted his normal or even accelerated progress with pride in the diary we kept. He was crawling by 6 months, standing up with support by $7\frac{1}{2}$ months, and walking by 9 months. Not long after that, he began to say his first words, and by 15 months he began stringing those words into sentences. He could also manipulate objects well, building tall towers of blocks and working simple inset puzzles. By 20 months of age he could identify letters, shapes, and colors, as well as recite parts of favorite books. Finally, we noticed that Jordan had an uncanny ability to pronounce words clearly and to sing simple songs on key.

Jordan's temperament during this period of his life was mostly even keel. He was not easily frustrated or opposed to changes. Though he expressed a clear preference for some activities over others, such as being read to and riding in the car, he did not seem compulsive about them.

Jordan's health at this time was also good, despite a fair number of ear infections that led to many doses of antibiotics and eventually to two operations in which tubes were inserted into his ears. These operations did not, however, seem to impact on his hearing, which has always seemed normal.

In short, Jordan was a jolly little guy who charmed and amused us all. Grandparents, aunts and uncles, friends, and the doctors who saw Jordan before he turned 2 had nothing but praise for his early development. The peculiarities he manifested, such as appearing to talk to himself and his fetish for rolling objects across the floor, were seen as minor quirks within a wholly normal development.

Shortly before he turned 2, though, certain aspects of Jordan's behavior began to change. Noises, like a vacuum cleaner or a motorcycle starting up, seemed to elicit inordinately fearful reactions. He developed periods of inexplicable negative responses to particular objects, situations, or people. He became obsessive about certain things, for example, asking to hear a favorite song over and over again. He also became less social and less interested in participating in structured activities. And finally, and most disconcertingly, he began to exhibit bizarre self-stimulatory behavior.

By the fall of 1984, we had come to the conclusion that Jordan was definitely different, and before Christmas of that year our concerns led us to seek medical help for answers. As with so many children who present cognitive, social, and communication deficiencies and yet have no sign of neurological injury, Jordan was eventually diagnosed as autistic or autistic-like. Though he certainly had many characteristics of this disorder, there was much about his early development and then-current functioning that didn't fit the pattern. Suspicions that we held about the medical profession's response to cases such as Jordan's were confirmed by the cursory brush-off we received when we tried to interest different physicians in the detailed diary that we kept of his first 2 years. Wasn't anyone interested in learning about this child who had changed so drastically for the worse without observable cause? There was a uniform and amazing lack of curiosity on the part of the professionals that to my mind could only be explained as disbelief of our story on their part. Interestingly enough, some of the other parents whose children are chronicled in this book have experienced the same reaction—even when they had videotape footage to prove their points. No wonder it has taken so long for even these beginning steps to be taken!

When the first round of medical reports was completed, we were then ready to have our day with the educational bureaucracy. Early in 1985, we visited one of the assessment sites for the Howard County, Maryland, public school system. By this time, Jordan was becoming increasingly difficult to keep on task, and we didn't have a lot of confidence that he would participate in the testing. He did, however, manage to minimally comply with most requests, though—being new to this business—we weren't sure that what was done in the session gave a true picture of what Jordan was capable of. Nevertheless, the assessment accomplished its main purpose, which was to qualify Jordan for special education services in the county's "early beginnings" program. The final results placed Jordan's cognitive functioning at about 6 months below age level on average and, in essence, confirmed what the earlier psychologist's reports had suggested—mild retardation.

The services Jordan received as a result of his diagnosis, although seriously inadequate to help a child with autism, were fairly standard for our area and perhaps for the rest of the country at the time. He qualified for two mornings a week in the early learning center where he received instruction with a couple of other children. He also received a visit from his teacher once a week, during which he experienced some of the same activities that were offered in school, and we were given advice as to how to reinforce what he was learning. In some ways, the whole program was rather mystifying, as his Individual Education Plan (IEP) called for instruction in concepts that he already knew, such as colors and shapes. But we were not fully aware of other options, such as the intense early intervention efforts suggested by Ivor Lovaas, that have helped some autistic children make remarkable recoveries, so we went along with the program.

Naturally, our ignorance of what a good plan might be to help Jordan didn't prevent us from taking a lot of action on our own, which we did consistently over the next year and a half. The first thing we tried to do to supplement the county's program was to conduct an altered behavior modification regimen at home, attempting to facilitate Jordan's improvement in language and concept development. Our efforts produced some positive early results. Jordan worked willingly and seemed to be getting the idea of spatial relationships, sequencing of events, and identifying categories. After about 6 weeks into the program, however, things began to deteriorate. He was no longer paying attention and was, in fact, actively seeking to avoid contact with everyone. He also began to sleep poorly, demand specific foods, and throw frequent temper tantrums. To make matters worse, he started to lose speech and cognitive abilities fairly rapidly.

This last development was not predicted by any of the professionals working with Jordan. Indeed, most of those who had tested or examined him suggested that his extensive vocabulary and fairly broad array of concepts would help to propel the social development necessary for further cognitive advances. No one, including us, expected Jordan to do what he actually did over the next few years, which was to virtually lose his humanity. The key to this process, which we now know in retrospect, was that Jordan mysteriously lost his ability and desire to cue into the signals and behavior of others as a source of learning. I later characterized this development as something akin to an astronaut becoming untethered on a spacewalk. Jordan drifted away helplessly, totally disconnected.

Like the other CDD families, we sought more desperate measures when traditional methods failed, among these being an intense, 14-hour-a-day, one-on-one therapy modeled after the program described in Barry Kaufman's book *Son Rise;* experiments with various drugs and vitamin supplements; and, finally, enrollment in Dr. Kiyo Kitahara's Tokyo Higashi School.

Our initial departure from the beaten path of therapy for Jordan came in the form of seeking a medical cure. We began this search sometime in the spring of 1985 after reading of promising results being achieved with persons suffering from autism using the drug fenfluramine. We had to go through many hoops to secure this drug—some of which went against the grain of our pediatrician, who likened our experimentation to child abuse. When fenfluramine proved inconsequential, we began to participate in a study on the drug naltrexone. Again, little impact on Jordan was noticed from this trial other than the stark terror he exhibited at having his blood drawn each time he received a dosage. At other times during this early period, we gave Jordan Ritalin, vitamin supplements, and DMG. We also, at various times, restricted or changed Jordan's diet to see if there was some allergic reaction in operation. None of these measures provided us with any clues or results.

As for our stint with the Kaufman program (which we did with Jordan from January to August 1986), we noticed no significant changes—aside from the continuing gradual decline in Jordan's spontaneous use of language. It would be difficult to assess what, if any, impact our constant attempts to make contact with him had during this period. My personal belief is that nothing would have been different in this regard even if we had tried methods that were diametrically opposed to those that we used.

Our failure, exhaustion, and need to return to full-time employment in the fall had led us to begin researching educational programs for autistic children during the spring of 1986. One name that kept coming up during this period was that of Dr. Kiyo Kitahara, principal and founder of the Tokyo Higashi School. The Higashi program offered autistic children the opportunity to go to school with normal peers, an idea that had particular appeal to Jill and me after our experiences with the isolated programs for special needs children in our county. There was the tremendous disadvantage of having to send Jordan to a residential school in a foreign country, where we would have very few opportunities to monitor his progress, but there seemed little to lose considering the fact that he appeared to be living on a foreign planet at the time anyway. All was settled in September, when we visited the school and came to the conclusion that our fear of losing control over Jordan was not as great as our desire to see him enrolled in a real school where he would have frequent contact with normal children, albeit ones who spoke Japanese.

Of all of the things that we tried with Jordan, the Higashi program seemed to have the most lasting effect. He remained in Tokyo for the duration of the 1986–1987 school year, returned as a residential student to Boston with the other American children in the program for the following 2 years, and then became a day student between 1989 and 1991. Jordan's tenure at Higashi resulted, we believe, in some noticeable improvements in his functioning. He slept through the night, became more responsive to directions, mastered most aspects of dressing and toileting, and developed better fine and gross motor skills. His receptive language may also have improved slightly, though his expressive language was—as it remains today—essentially gone. The Higashi personnel were also instrumental in getting us to work harder with Jordan and to view him more positively. They were willing to work long hours with him and demonstrated on many occasions a kindness toward and appreciation of him that touched us deeply.

In July 1991, we decided to return to Maryland. The overriding consideration in that decision was the belief that a more stable financial picture would enable our entire family to have a happier life, but we also had come to the conclusion that the Higashi program had done all that could be expected of it.

Our 5-year association with the Higashi school was, as I indicated, a mostly positive experience. The kind of instruction Dr. Kitahara recommended, namely, vigorous physical exercise, learning through the arts, and mixed education with normal peers (what we now call inclusion), had much to offer a child like Jordan. And seeing the Higashi teachers in action as we did in September 1986 gave us great confidence. As did the comments of parents whose children had been at the school the year before. And, finally, the inevitability of a U.S. branch of Higashi opening in Boston for the 1987–1988 school year pushed us over the edge. It was a momentous decision to leave a little child halfway around the world and to sign a check for $25,000 to pay for it, but we never had second thoughts.

Having visited Jordan only twice during his first year at Higashi, we had little to go on regarding his progress. The school did call us occasionally, and they also sent a monthly tape of the activities that he had been participating in, though they were very short and carefully edited. We could ascertain from the films some definite trends, however, most notably that Jordan had better eye contact and was following directions readily. When he returned home for summer vacation—along with a live-in teacher from the school—we began to realize that the things he had been doing for his teachers were not immediately transferable to us. While in the company of the teacher, he was calm and more attentive, but with us he was his old hyper and unfocused self. Nothing we saw during the vacation, however, caused us to doubt our decision to have Jordan remain a student there.

Marginal improvement in his capabilities continued over the next 2 years, and by the spring of 1989 Jill and I began to agree with the school's administration that Jordan should become a day student. By this time, Maryland had begun funding Jordan's placement at Higashi, and we anticipated few problems with continuing the funding when we moved to Massachusetts, especially as Jordan was going to be moving from a residential to a day placement. Things really looked settled when—in an act of extraordinary compassion—the Maryland Attorney General's Office consented to allowing Jill to work part time in Maryland and part time in Massachusetts. The deal became complete when my inlaws agreed to allow Jill and Leslie to stay with them during those weeks when she would be back in Maryland. The long-term plan called for me to get a job in Massachusetts and for Jill to eventually get admitted to the Massachusetts bar.

The first year of this arrangement was quite difficult. The monthly 2-week separation from Jill and Leslie, my inability to find a teaching job, and the onerous adjustment to living with an autistic child again made things seem as if they would fall apart. But a break occurred in July 1990 when the Higashi school administration offered me a job as director of development, and Jill began to position herself for a special education law practice.

The auspicious start to the final year, however, didn't last long. Increasingly, Jordan was becoming aggressive and self-injurious. There were numerous instances in which teachers, bus drivers, respite work-ers, and even family members fell victim to Jordan's rage. Particularly in the mornings, he seemed unsettled and unpredictable. Some of the episodes of that time were especially scary, and, for a time, we began to question the practices of the school. We wondered whether the de-manding regimen of the instructional program might be causing his frustration. We also began to question our ability to make it financially when Jill officially severed her ties with the Attorney General's Office, an intuition that seemed increasingly accurate when Jill's practice failed to bring in the expected income.

A culmination of many factors finally swayed us in the direction of returning to Maryland by the spring of 1991, not the least of which were the realities of full-time employment opportunities awaiting both Jill and me when we returned. Jill was offered a job as counsel to Mary-land's governor, and I was rehired by Baltimore's school system as an el-ementary school assistant principal. Having the time to investigate options for Jordan, we were also able to enroll him in a public school autism program about which we felt very confident. Montgomery County, one of Maryland's richest jurisdictions, had been developing this program for autistic children for a number of years and now had sites up and running within several of their public elementary schools. Jordan would now have the opportunity to be around normal peers for a good part of his day.

In the spring of 1991, we spent a few days house hunting and came up with a place situated in a neighborhood close to good schools for both Leslie and Jordan. Settlement was reached in early summer. We moved in in August and began to recapture some forward mo-mentum in our lives. Though we were able to return to some sem-blance of normalcy, things didn't immediately improve for us. To start, Jordan continued to display very erratic behavior, though the worst elements of his aggression did seem to abate. Now 9 years old, he presented new challenges. His increased size, although remaining normal in appearance, made it more difficult for others not familiar with the behavior of such a child to understand and excuse his bizarre actions. Trips to the store were and remain to this day a source of ad-venture. Frequently, he would take things off of the shelves, knock down displays, touch strangers inappropriately, and jump up and down making loud noises.

His unpredictability made me very nervous. Although some of his behavior had obvious antecedents, you could never be sure that he wasn't going to create a huge scene out of the blue. On one occasion, he approached a teenage boy in a parking lot and spit in his face. Fortunately, the young fellow was quite understanding. Many other folks, however, weren't quite as nice, and often I found myself torn between wanting to apologize for Jordan and fighting the urge to lash out at someone for being insensitive over a minor affront or inconvenience.

Another aspect of Jordan's behavior that changed as he got older was his tendency to disappear if he wasn't carefully watched. Occasionally, this led to situations where serious consequences could have resulted. For example, about a year after we had moved in, we established a regular walking route around the neighborhood. One day we were about to embark on that daily constitutional when the phone rang. As Jordan had always waited patiently during such interruptions, I gave no second thought to answering the phone. On this particular day, however, Jordan decided that he didn't need a partner for the walk and went off on his own, a decision that might have had tragic consequences, as he still could not be counted on to avoid cars. After getting off the phone, I immediately looked for Jordan in the backyard, where he normally waited. Not finding him right away, I realized what must have happened and took off on a dead run along our usual path. I caught up with him several minutes later and finally spotted him swinging in a tree about half a mile away from home.

On another occasion, Jordan got out of my sight in a grocery store when I had become preoccupied in a conversation with a neighbor. When I caught up with him this time, he was hanging on the cart barrier in the front of the store. Incidents such as these have made me almost obsessively insistent on Jordan's staying right beside me whenever we are out. And this overprotectiveness has been viewed at times—like a normal child would see it—as suffocating by Jordan.

About the time that we came back to Maryland, Jordan also began to develop greater social awareness and interest. Sometimes this new behavior was a source of excitement and joy, such as when he would come and join us in bed at night before everyone went to sleep, or when he spontaneously hugged us. At other times, though, this trait caused problems, like when Jordan would purposefully take toys from or otherwise tease his sister. We were hopeful that Jordan's increased social sense would help us open doors for him in the community. Toward that end, we enrolled him in summer camps and recreational programs, realizing, at best, mixed results. On the one hand, he got to associate with normal peers and to participate in activities that were age appropriate and fun. On the other hand, he was frequently sent home from these adventures because the companions assigned to him weren't able to keep him sufficiently under control.

This problem of inadequately prepared staff was not confined to summer camps. As Jordan got older and stronger, his erratic behavior often presented challenges to the after-school and respite care personnel as well. Jordan wasn't typical of the clientele such groups serve. Unlike the compliant, mildly retarded children and young adults in these programs, Jordan showed no interest in the simple tabletop activities, video programs, and field trips that were provided. Moreover, the staff was usually comprised of high school students or recent graduates with little or no experience. Not knowing how to involve Jordan in the group activities, their reactions alternated between benign neglect and overly aggressive attempts to get him involved.

For the first 2 years in which we lived in Maryland, this problem was only an annoyance. But it nearly became a crisis in the spring of 1994 when the only after-school program serving autistic children in our area informed us that Jordan could not return to their program in the fall. At this same time, we were experiencing difficulty keeping respite workers. The situation was a significant departure from our experience in Massachusetts where, first of all, a block of respite time was provided free of charge by the state, and second, we had more time to take Jordan ourselves because of our reduced work schedules. A third factor that made life a little easier in Massachusetts in this regard was the availability of the Higashi personnel in the event of a crisis.

In our new circumstances, the lack of after-school care and diminished respite services was more than an inconvenience; it meant that somehow we would have to come up with a workable plan for Jordan's care after school and for weekends. Though it was draining, particularly during the winter months, we could handle the weekend times on our own. But getting reliable coverage during the week would be another matter. Initially, we considered hiring a regular baby-sitter, or a team of them, but our experience with individuals willing to baby-sit for Jordan had been that there was little assurance that any such sitter would be dependable, especially after seeing how difficult Jordan could be to handle. It was looking more and more that I would simply leave my job and take care of him myself.

As if by divine intervention, however, we learned of Maryland's Systems Reform Initiative (SRI) from the supervisor of the Montgomery County Autism program just days after the end of the school year. The purpose of this program is to maintain "at-risk" students in home placements by providing the additional services that would make it possible for their families to keep them at home. Shortly after we applied to this program, the Local Coordinating Council (the entity that decides eligibility for these services) scheduled us for a meeting to determine if we would qualify.

Within a matter of days after the hearing, our application for services was approved. We were assigned a caseworker who facilitated our getting additional weekend and evening respite as well as began reviewing options for after-school respite in the fall. Further good luck befell us when we learned of Troy Marbly's interest in working with Jordan after school. Troy had been one of Jordan's teachers for the past several years and had been working on a number of initiatives to help Jordan increase self-help and communication skills. As Troy was with Jordan on a daily basis, this arrangement would be like a natural extension of his school program. And it would be carried out in settings that varied from Troy's own home to various places in the community.

Over the past 2½ years, this program has been nothing short of a miracle. Not only has Jordan benefited from Troy's additional involvement—becoming like a member of his family—but he has also received the opportunity to do many quality things in the community as a result of the additional respite and recreational programs that are provided for with SRI. And, though not cheap, I am certain that the program has been cost effective for the state of Maryland in that Jordan would almost certainly have been found eligible for a residential placement had not the additional services been available.

The changes that SRI has wrought in the lives of the rest of our family have been equally significant. For the first time, Jill and I were able to attend Leslie's school and athletic events together. It also became easier for Leslie to have friends over, though she has always been—amazingly to us—very matter-of-fact and reassuring regarding her brother's odd behavior with those friends. Simple things like eating out were also returned to our lives. There was even a noticeable effect on our careers. Instead of one or both of us drastically curtailing or even quitting our jobs, we both were able to take positions of greater responsibility. Jill continued with her application and was successful in landing a job as a federal magistrate judge, and I became a principal of a school. Assuming these positions would have been unthinkable before SRI.

Despite the wonderful assistance we have received over the past 3 years through our association with the many organizations that have become involved with Jordan's life, the challenges of caring for an adolescent with CDD/autism remain daunting. A willful person, in a strong and nearly adult frame, with normal reaction time and limited communication and self-help skills presents ongoing problems. Constant vigilance is required to ensure his safety, especially as his favorite activity involves placing his body at risk for falling from the tops of steps and playground equipment. In the past 3 years, he has fallen down the steps leading from our kitchen to the basement dozens of times, and he has also fallen from the upstairs steps—a much more dangerous trip—at least 10 times. No bones have been broken in these escapades, but one of his permanent teeth has been cracked and rebroken on at least 2 occasions. Trying to prevent him from doing this has only resulted in huge frustration on his part, as he doesn't associate the activity with the consequences, or he simply is so driven to seek this thrill that he can't be reasonably controlled.

Though less frightening, the challenge of trying to keep Jordan occupied may be even more draining. He does not enjoy any activity, aside from eating, sleeping, step swinging, and autoerotic play. An evening with Jordan typically involves dinner, a bath, and vain attempts to develop primitive leisure skills. There was a time, before adolescence, when we could distract and cajole him into nearly an hour's worth of semiproductive time every evening. But his increased size and willfulness have made this undertaking less and less successful over time. Surprisingly, Leslie has maintained greater power over Jordan in this regard and can still get him to do an occasional puzzle, but Jordan has always found Leslie much more interesting than us.

Although Jordan is more manageable at school, some diminution in his cooperativeness has been observed there as well. As if to say to all of us, "Hey, adolescent rebelliousness is a part of everyone's life: Live with it!" Jordan has found new ways to get under the skin of his teachers. His method of choice to show his disdain for those who would try to structure his behavior is to make loud noises or laugh in their faces or to grab hold of their hands, an act that can be particularly annoying given his surprising hand strength. And grabbing someone's hands when they are driving the car has a particular attraction for Jordan, even when he is placed in the back seat.

In a couple of days, Jordan will turn 15 years old. He has grown so rapidly over the past 18 months that virtually none of the clothes that he wore 2 years ago fit. For a normal child, this growth might be an interesting aside to the more complex social, emotional, and intellectual development that adolescents undergo. But for Jordan, it is the sole significant change. The mute, isolated toddler that he became with the onset of autism/CDD over 12 years ago has merely taken up new residence in this newly enlarged frame. It reminds me of the descriptions of how the universe is said to have begun—a singularity that has expanded, creating the increased space but retaining its original material. It is difficult to capture the surreal quality of these physical changes taking place in a person in the absence of the expected mental development.

As time has elapsed, and our daughter has grown older and more of a companion to us, Jill and I have found ourselves increasingly involved in her life and decreasingly involved in Jordan's. Soccer, swimming, camps, band concerts, homework—the stuff of normal childhood—have become our agenda as well. Games won or lost, boys crashing her birthday party, performances in plays, the death of a pet—the things that give a life a story—have evolved and deepened around Leslie's existence. The dots can't be drawn together so easily for Jordan. On New Year's Day this year Jordan and I went to the grocery store. The lines were long and it was well past our usual lunch hour. Each customer preceding us seemed to have a particular problem that required additional time to resolve. As the last person ahead of us began to place his items on the counter, I heard a low growl—almost like a dog's—coming from behind. I turned to see Jordan grimacing as if in great pain. Before I could get to and try to comfort him, he began to strike his head with closed fists and to emit a terrible wail. I knew that a very unpleasant scene was about to take place, so I tried to convince Jordan to walk calmly outside with me to the car. But he would have nothing of it. Instead, he lashed out with his fists at me. I moved toward the exit as quickly and unobtrusively as was possible with Jordan pursuing and hitting—alternately me and himself—as we left the store. In the parking lot, he continued to howl and strike himself. He also ran out into the path of the cars, which were—fortunately—not going very fast. After a brief struggle, I finally got him into the car and out onto the road going home. As we drove, Jordan continued to scream and strike both me and himself. I tried to get him to stop with different methods, including striking him back, but he wouldn't calm down until we were almost home.

At home, he whimpered and greedily ate the lunch I hastily prepared and then went to rest in his bed. Later that afternoon, Leslie and Jill returned from an outing. Jill heard me describe what had happened and went to engage Jordan to see if she could comfort him. But this just aggravated Jordan further, and he became involved in escalating aggression toward her. It was hours before the whole agonizing business had settled down. That night in bed I was reminded of a New Year's Day 13 years ago—ironically, 1984—when we had received a phone call informing us of the death of a close friend. At the time, I had thought to myself, "What an awful way to start the new year, I hope it isn't a harbinger of things to come." It was in December of that year that we learned of Jordan's diagnosis. Would history be repeating itself?

The next few days were ones of great soul-searching for Jill and me. Though we saw Jordan less frequently these days because of all of the respite we were given, we were also less and less able to handle some of these down moments. Additionally, we had become increasingly afraid that these kinds of encounters we had every so often with Jordan were frightening to Leslie. She is a sharp and understanding child, but repeated exposures to inexplicable outbursts where nothing a parent does seems to be able to settle a sibling can't help but have psychological consequences, or so we have come to believe.

We were in the beginning stages of wondering whether a residential placement might not be a reality to come sooner than later. At first it was just a thought. After all, Jordan had not deteriorated significantly at school, and there had really been no discussion of such a placement among the players planning his educational program. But during the first few weeks at school after the holiday Jordan was showing signs of being less manageable. Notes from his teacher indicated that he laughed inappropriately more frequently and that he had become more confrontational. And he continued to have some problems at home. Maybe it was time to at least broach the subject with his teachers and other caretakers.

When we actually took the initiative to bring our concerns to Kris Secan, the autism coordinator for Montgomery County Schools, we were surprised to hear that she and others who had worked with Jordan had wondered why we hadn't pressed for this kind of placement earlier. Her caring and cooperative attitude had always been a blessing to us, but never more so than when we had to make this difficult decision. Jordan's teacher, Terry Scott, concurred with Kris and offered to support our efforts to secure the placement. As did Troy Marbly and Margie Lidoff, Jordan's SRI caseworker. So complete was the agreement that when our placement hearing was held there was little discussion but for the details of the transition.

In April of this year, Jordan started in a group home run by the Grafton School. He is residential in their program but remains a day student in the Montgomery County public schools. All of the parties that worked with Jordan prior to his placement continue to work with him now, and this is a key to the successful start that he has enjoyed. It is an immeasurable comfort to know that Jordan is only a 10-minute drive away, that we can have access to him at any time, and that skilled and caring people are working with him around the clock. It is also reassuring to know that Jordan gets time in the community and has an educational program that is structured beyond the daytime hours.

Each weekend since his placement he has spent some time at home, and already we are seeing subtle changes in his behavior. One significant and definite change is that he has attempted to initiate communication on his own. It hasn't been a huge and dramatic advance in this regard, but it represents the kind of incremental steps that a full-time organized program can offer a significantly handicapped person. By placing such a person in a situation that makes more demands of him, growth is far more likely to occur—a circumstance we take for granted with normal people.

It's certainly too early in this experience to say that the river will run peacefully from here on in. We, as all parents, have learned not to expect the unreasonable. But the latest bend in the river has brought new vistas we had not thought possible—for us and for Jordan.

Author Biographies

Kjell Berg is a 47-year-old civil engineer working with technical information. His wife is a teacher. They have a 14-year-old daughter and a 10-year-old son, Per, about whom their chapter is written. The Berg family lives in a little town, Ljungby, in southern Sweden.

Sheila Brown is married to Stewart, and they have four children between the ages of 16 years and 6 months. They live on a sheep and cattle farm in the center of the North Island of New Zealand. Sheila was born in England, where she gained an honors degree in biology and became a high school teacher. She has been living in New Zealand for nearly 20 years.

Madeline Catalano is a speech/language therapist who has taught children with various disabilities, including autism. She is a graduate of SUNY at Albany and received a master of science in education degree from the College of St. Rose in Albany, New York. She participates in telephone counseling of parents of autistic children for Parent Network of Buffalo, New York, as well as in counseling parents of children with CDD. She lives in Portville, New York, with her husband Robert (editor of *When Autism Strikes*) and children Chris, Ruth, Thomas, and Matthew.

Marie Day is a pseudonym. She is a volunteer at the local Learning Assistant Program, which is geared to help children and adults improve their reading skills. She resides in Canada with her husband and four children.

Jenny Fairthorne is a secondary mathematics teacher. Her husband Fred is a grocery retailer. They have three children, Tom, Sarah, and David, about whom her chapter is written. Recently, David's zest for life has been further buoyed by his massive progress in signed communication. The Fairthorne family lives in Nedlands in suburban Perth, western Australia.

Stephen Ferris works as a public servant in the Department of Foreign Affairs and Trade. *Sue Ferris* has worked in the home since having three children—Mark (8), Laura (7), and Joanna (5). The Ferris family has recently moved from Canberra, Australia, to Tasmania. This move has enabled Laura to attend a school specializing in teaching autistic children and was a necessity since Laura had regressed in her Canberra school. The family hopes to move back to Canberra if appropriate education becomes available to Laura there.

Candice Goldstein lives with her husband, Abraham Steinberg, a urologist, and their two children in Geneva, Illinois, a Chicago suburb. She is a graduate of the University of Michigan and the University of Illinois College of Law. She edits *Bad Faith Law Update*, a monthly legal publication, from home.

Craig Schulze is a school administrator specializing in curriculum for the Baltimore, Maryland, school system. For the past 10 years he has written articles on education for *The Baltimore Sun*, *The Evening Sun*, and *Middlesex News*. In 1993, Woodbine House Publishers published Schulze's book *When Snow Turns to Rain*—a chronicle of his family's experiences raising an autistic son. Craig is a graduate of Western Maryland College and has received a Ph.D. from the University of Maryland in human development. He serves on the board of directors for the Montgomery County Autism Society.

Index

239

Support networks
  Allergy-Induced Autism Support and
    Research Network, 188
  CAN (Cure Autism Now) International,
    188
  CANDLE (childhood aphasia, neuro-
    logical disorders, Landau-Kleffner,
    and epilepsy), 122
  Developmental Delay Registry, 188–
    189
  importance of, 188
  international CDD network, 53, 141–
    144
  Landau-Kleffner syndrome (LKS), fami-
    lies of sufferers, 113
Sweden, 1–11
Swimming, 7, 140
Systems Reform Initiative (SRI)
  Maryland, 232, 236

Tantrums
  Catalano, Thomas, 38
  Ferris, Laura, 163, 171–172, 175, 182
TEACH (Treatment and Education of
    Autistic and Related Communica-
    tion Handicapped Children), 170
Tegretol, 84
Tender, Jura, 108
Thimerosal, 180
"Thomas the Tank Engine" (cartoon),
    196
Thompson, Helen, 106–108
Thomson, Rosalind, 106
Toilet training
  Berg, Per, 2
  Catalano, Thomas, 40
  Fairthorne, David, 115
  Ferris, Laura, 180–181
  Goldstein, Ben, 195
Tokyo, University of, 168
Tokyo Higashi School, 226–228, 231
Tom and Pippo (Oxenbury), 93, 101
Tumbling Tots program, 201, 204

Ultrasound, 170
United Kingdom, 25
United States, 191–236
Utah State University, 179

Vaccinations
  Fairthorne, David, 92, 137

Vaccinations (cont.)
  Ferris, Laura, 168–169, 173, 176, 178,
    180, 181, 183, 186, 187
  Goldstein, Ben, 193
  Van Slyke, Pat, 199–201, 203
Very Hungry Caterpillar, 106, 139
Video monitoring, 126
Vigabratin, 125, 128
Violin playing, 96, 98, 110
Vitamin and mineral supplements
  Brown, Nicky ("Pickle"), 23–24
  Catalano, Thomas, 48–49
  Ferris, Laura, 177–178
  Goldstein, Ben, 214
Volkmar, Fred R., vii-ix, 52–53
  Fairthorne family and, 114–116, 118,
    133, 137, 141
  Ferris family and, 168
  international CDD network and, 141,
    144

Walking, early, 2, 70
Wall, Martin, 99, 120
Walsh, Dr., 141
  EEG, 150, 158
  epileptic regression, 125
  first meeting with, 111
  Landau-Kleffner syndrome (LKS), test-
    ing for, 113–114, 146–147
  MRI, discussion on, 117
  Princess Margaret Hospital, examina-
    tion, 122
Waring, Rosemary, 152, 177
Warren, Reed, 179
Weinum, Tracey, 204
Wetting, 219–220
Wheaton College, 205–206
When Snow Turns to Rain (Schulze), 53,
    222, 223, 238
Wise, Grahame, 117, 119–121
Woodall, Harold, 105
Woods, Sally, 99–100

X syndrome, fragile, 121

Yale University, 114
Yeast-related autism, 49
Young Autism Project (Murdoch Univer-
    sity), 108, 147

Zoloft, 56, 213–214